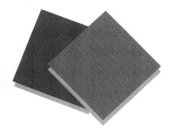

AUTOETHNOGRAPHY AS METHOD

Developing Qualitative Inquiry
Series Editor:
Janice Morse,
University of Utah

Books in the new *Developing Qualitative Inquiry* series, written by leaders in qualitative inquiry, will address important topics in qualitative methods. Targeted to a broad multidisciplinary readership, the books are intended for mid-level/advanced researchers and advanced students. The series will forward the field of qualitative inquiry by describing new methods or developing particular aspects of established methods. Proposals for the series should be sent to the series editor at explore@LCoastPress.com.

Volumes in this series:
Autoethnography as Method, Heewon Chang

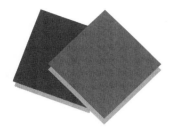

AUTOETHNOGRAPHY
AS METHOD

Heewon Chang

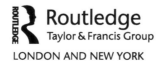

Routledge
Taylor & Francis Group

LONDON AND NEW YORK

First published 2008 by Left Coast Press, Inc.

Published 2016 by Routledge
2 Park Square, Milton Park, Abingdon, Oxon OX14 4RN
52 Vanderbilt Avenue, New York, NY 10017

Routledge is an imprint of the Taylor & Francis Group, an informa business

Library of Congress Cataloging-in-Publication Data:

Chang, Heewon, 1959-
Autoethnography as method/Heewon Chang.
    p. cm. — (Developing qualitative inquiry)
Includes bibliographical references and index.
   ISBN 978-1-59874-122-3 (hardback : alk. paper)
   ISBN 978-1-59874-123-0 (pbk. : alk. paper)
1. Ethnology—Biographical methods. 2. Autobiography. 3. Ethnology—Authorship.
4. Ethnology—Field work. I. Title.
   GN346.6.C53 2008   305.8—dc22   2007044268

ISBN 13: 978-1-59874-122-3 (hbk)
ISBN 13: 978-1-59874-123-0 (pbk)

CONTENTS

To the many "edgewalkers" in my life,
Especially Klaus, Hannah, and Peter,
Who are always willing to take a risk of embracing novelty

To my *Doktorvater*, mentor, friend, and colleague
Harry
Who has believed in me

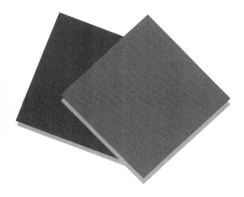

PREFACE

Over a delicious, yet simple, meal served by nuns in Säben, a cloister located in Northern Italy, my German sister-in-law asked what I had been up to lately. My answer, "I'm writing a book," obviously piqued her curiosity. Instead of taunting me for working during a mini-family reunion at that peaceful locale, she immediately tossed her second question at me, "What is it about?"

Without hesitation I replied, "It's about autoethnography." She then wondered aloud if I was too young to write an autobiography. She obviously caught the "auto" portion in my answer. I could tell that she was assuming that autoethnography had something to do with autobiography. Her reasoning is acceptable, provided that a life is still forming for a person of my age and that no complete personal history could ever be written so early. Although she was partially correct in her assumption, I felt compelled to clarify further. I explained that my book is not about my autobiography per se, but about a research method that utilizes the researchers' autobiographical data to analyze and interpret their cultural assumptions. This explanation was lofty and abstract. Instead of pursuing it further, my sister-in-law dropped the subject and moved on to a more engaging topic for conversation. How could I have described the book better to my sister-in-law?

Now I face the same challenge of describing my book, this time, to a different audience—experienced and novice researchers who may or may not be convinced that personal stories can mix well with scholarship. Fortunately, I am not a lone voice in the wilderness, who proclaims there is a way of integrating the personal into academics. Others such as Anderson (2006), Ellis and Bochner (2000), Nash (2004), Reed-Danahay (1997), and Tompkins (1996) have already plowed through the wilderness to make a path, and many have followed them. Yet, I still smell fresh-cut grass along the trail and have felt an urge to show my students and interested others one more way of utilizing personal stories for scholarly purposes. So I have decided to write a book grounded in the anthropological tradition of ethnography and a hands-on approach to instruction in research methods.

These three distinctive characteristics—anthropological, methodological, and practical—are embedded in both the structure and the content of the book. This book is divided into three parts and presents six appendices. Part I presents three conceptual chapters that address in turn the concepts of culture, the tradition of self-narratives, and the development of autoethnography. In this part, the concept of culture is discussed from an anthropological perspective, and autoethnography is affirmed as an ethnographic research method that focuses on cultural analysis and interpretation.

Part II contains one introductory chapter and three methodology chapters to guide data collection in autoethnographic "fieldwork." Chapter 4 introduces the very first step of research—"getting ready" with research topics, research design, and ethical consideration. Focusing on personal memory data, self-observational and self-reflective data, and external data, Chapters 5 through 7 introduce practical data collection strategies and writing exercises to aid data collection. The writing exercises and corresponding writing samples of mine are compiled in Appendix A. You may adopt them to stimulate your data collection process. However, I encourage you to expand them to fit your research purpose.

Part III presents additional methodological chapters. These three chapters suggest a variety of practical strategies of data management, data analysis and interpretation, and autoethnographic writing. The chapters in Part III are critical in the autoethnographic process because the activities suggested will ultimately shape data into autoethnography and give an ethnographic flavor to this research inquiry. Please note that I will adopt a more academic writing style in Part I and a more informal one in Parts II and III. Through this informal style, I hope to bring research to a comfortable level for all readers.

Every piece of writing reflects the disposition of its author. This book is not an exception; it subtly and explicitly reveals who I am and what I value. It represents my professional interest in anthropology, education, multicultural education, ethnography, and self-narratives.

Intermingled with these is my personal fascination with self-reflection, introspection, intrapersonal intelligence, and self-analysis. My faith—particularly focusing on "hospitality for strangers" (Pohl, 1999) and love of neighbors—has also laid groundwork for my thinking. These professional and personal interests of mine are likely to be building blocks of this book. They may show up in my suggested writing exercises; strategies of data collection, analysis, and interpretation; and writing samples.

None of these exercises is intended as the authoritative and prescriptive way of completing an autoethnography. Rather, they should be seen as suggestions coming from a person who has been experimenting with this relatively new ethnographic method for a while. Thus, I invite you to look into the world of my biases and experiences, take whatever is useful, and discard what does not fit your needs.

Authors are not solitary creators of their work; rather, their works are products of caring, nurturing, and supportive communities of constructive critiques. I am deeply indebted to many colleagues, mentors, and authors as well as family members and friends who have opened doors to their hearts and minds throughout my life. It is impossible to name them all here. With a deep sense of inadequacy in acknowledging all by name, I have to be content with some who have been instrumental in shaping this book.

I am immensely grateful to Dr. Harry Wolcott, my *Doktorvater* (a German word for a doctoral advisor who often becomes a lifelong mentor like a parent) from the University of Oregon, who has continued to serve as a mentor for a quarter of a century; Dr. Linda Stine, my friendly neighbor and personal editor, whose encouragement and support are bottomless; Dr. Mitch Allen and Dr. Janice Morse, my publisher and my editor from Left Coast Press, who have believed in my work; Dr. Geoffrey Walford, whose encouragement to publish an article on autoethnography affirmed my thinking and accelerated the progress of this book; Dr. Letty Lincoln, my colleague from the University of Oregon, who has always rendered supportive and constructive critiques; Dr. Soon Yong Park, Dr. Kum Yong Whang, Dr. Sang Jin Kang, and Dr. Myung Kun Lee, colleagues from Yonsei University in Seoul, Korea, who generously embraced the idea of a workshop on autoethnography and made it happen on their campus in the summer of 2006; and Dr. Jaime J. Romo and the University of North Carolina Press for allowing me to reprint his autoethnography in Appendix F.

Assistance from Eastern University came in many ways. Without the university's gift of time and financial support during my sabbatical year in 2005–2006, I would not have been able to carve out a chunk of time to sit down and write. I also want to acknowledge my former Dean, Dr. Vivian Nix-Early, who champions faculty causes, and colleagues from the Education Department—Dr. Helen Loeb, Dr. Dorothy Hurley, Dr. William Yerger, Dr. Jean Landis, Dr. Kathy-Ann Hernandez, Ms. Sue Seltzer, Ms. Sue Shaw, Ms. Adele Ressler, and Mr. Jim Osborne—who carried on with multiple responsibilities to cover for me during my absence. In addition, a special mention is due to Judy Ha and Reeja Koshy, confident graduate students from Eastern University, who helped compile the bibliography of self-narratives and thoroughly checked the accuracy of references, respectively.

Families of authors are often shortchanged during book making. My husband, Klaus Volpert, has been a constant supporter who understands the pressure in academia so well, who applauds my success before anyone, and who created time and space for me to write even during our family vacation. Blessed with the patient understanding of my two children, Hannah and Peter, I'm really a lucky parent. I also extend my deepest gratitude to my parents Chin-Ho Chang and Eui-Sook Cho, who have instilled in me the love of learning, believing, and caring; my parents-in-law Helmut and Waltraud Volpert, who have modeled cross-cultural and cross-religious acceptance; and to my sisters and sisters-in-law, Hee-Young, Hee-Eun, Hee-Bong, Ulrike, Maria, and Elisabeth, who have affirmed the strength of girl power for me.

All these individuals have helped me become who I am and, in turn, have contributed to this book in both big and small ways. Yet, I must assume sole responsibility for the content of the book, as a painter does for her painting. Others have inspired me, provided for me, critiqued my work, and sometimes suggested better brush strokes. All these helpers have made the book a better product. Now it is about time for me to put my signature on the painting and claim responsibility as its creator.

May 2007
Wayne, PA
USA

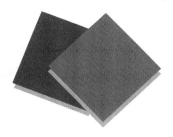

PART I
Conceptual Framework

Consisting of three chapters, Part I lays out the conceptual framework of the book, which is grounded on four assumptions: (1) culture is a group-oriented concept by which self is always connected with others; (2) the reading and writing of self-narratives provides a window through which self and others can be examined and understood; (3) telling one's story does not automatically result in the *cultural* understanding of self and others, which only grows out of in-depth cultural analysis and interpretation; and (4) autoethnography is an excellent instructional tool to help not only social scientists but also practitioners—such as teachers, medical personnel, counselors, and human services workers—gain profound understanding of self and others and function more effectively with others from diverse cultural backgrounds.

Chapter 1 elaborates on the concept of culture as a web of self and others. In this chapter, three elements—culture, self, and others—are explored in depth. Following the introduction of multiple perspectives on culture, the concepts of self and others are discussed. In Chapter 2, given the heightened interest in self-narratives in the social sciences, I argue that self-narratives can be used as cultural texts through which the cultural understanding of self and others can be gained. A variety of self-narratives are introduced and discussed in terms of genre, authorship, thematic focus, and writing style. Finally, in Chapter 3, autoethnography is singled out from among the many self-narrative varieties and compared and contrasted with other types of self-narratives. Readers will learn about the benefits of this research method as well as pitfalls to avoid when they adopt autoethnography as a research method. Readers who prefer to delve immediately into methodology may skip Part I and go directly to Part II.

Culture: A Web of Self and Others

The concept of culture fundamentally affects how we conduct a cultural study. It shapes our research questions, our sources of data, our analysis/interpretation, and our writing. So it is appropriate to begin this research guidebook with a discussion of the concept of culture. Since anthropologists invented the notion of culture, innumerable definitions and concepts have entered the literature of anthropology. My intention in this chapter is not to provide a comprehensive list of definitions, but to focus on concepts of culture that address people as interactive agents. After introducing various perspectives on the locus of culture—where culture resides—I shift my focus of discussion to "self," and then "others," both vital agents and participants in culture.

The Concepts of Culture

"I'm a typical American just like everyone else in this room," a student of mine proclaimed with an air of certainty in her voice. Without flinching, another student declared that her "individual culture" represents who she is. These are common statements that I hear from students of multicultural education when they are asked to define themselves culturally. Whether these statements accurately convey the meaning of "culture" will be discussed later. These statements represent two perspectives on culture. The first student's view associates culture with a group of people, in this case, Americans. Her statement implies that there is a definable American culture that she shares with other "Americans" who are identified by clear boundaries. Typical assumed boundaries for culture include nationality, ethnicity, language, and geography. In this case, she selected nationality and geographic boundaries to define her own people as "everyone else in this [American college class] room."

On the other hand, the second student considers culture from an individual's point of view. To her, the definition of culture begins with her. Her belief, behaviors, and perspective define who she is. She does not articulate how her "individual culture" overlaps with others and how different her individual culture is from others. Despite her lack of attention to relationships with others in the society, her focus on individuals draws our attention to the fact that people are neither blind followers of a predefined set of social norms, cultural clones of their previous generations, nor copycats of their cultural contemporaries. Rather, her perspective implies that individuals have autonomy to interpret and alter cultural knowledge and skills acquired from others and to develop their own version of culture while staying in touch with social expectations.

These two different perspectives of culture pursue answers to the same question that anthropologists have asked for over a century: "Where is culture located?" De Munck (2000) expands the question: Is culture located "out there, in the public world" or "in here, in the private sphere of the self"? The question of cultural locus may inadvertently associate culture with something tangible to locate. This association is not intended at all. Although defining culture is a tricky business in our contemporary, complex society, as Agar (2006) agonizes, I do not relegate culture to the physical realm of cultural artifacts. Before delving into what I mean by culture, however, I will discuss how anthropologists have tried to answer this locus question because their answers have important implications for the later discussion of autoethnography.

Symbiosis of Culture and People

First, I need to establish a nonnegotiable premise: the concept of culture is inherently group-oriented, because culture results from human interactions with each other. The notion of "individual culture" does not, and should not, imply that culture is about the psychological workings of an isolated individual; rather, it refers to individual versions of group cultures that are formed, shared, retained, altered, and sometimes shed through human interactions. These interactions may take place in "local communities of practice" in which "what particular persons do [is] in mutual influence upon one another as they associate regularly together" (Erickson, 2004, p. 38). Gajjala (2004) would argue that face-to-face interactions are not a prerequisite to the creation of culture in a highly globalized digital age when interactions can be facilitated by digital means of communication—such as e-mail, telephone, and the Internet. Her cyber-ethnographic study of listservs for South Asian professional women demonstrates that a cyber cultural community can be formed and undergo a transformation into something that is similar to a local cultural community. Whether interactions are conventional or alternative, the fundamental premise that culture has something to do with human interactions within a group is not challenged.

De Munck (2000) expresses the symbiotic relationship between culture and people as follows:

> Obviously, one does not exist as a psyche—a self—outside of culture; nor does culture exist independently of its bearers. . . . Culture would cease to exist without the individuals who make it up. . . . Culture requires our presence as individuals. With this symbiosis, self and culture together make each other up and, in that process, make meaning. (pp. 1–2)

Resonating with this perspective, Rosaldo (1984) declares that we "are not individuals first but social persons" (p. 151).

Although the premise that culture and people are intertwined may be indisputable, it does not produce an equally unequivocal answer to the question: "Where is culture located?" This question has been entertained since the beginning of anthropology as an academic discipline, and answers are divided into two groups: one argues that culture is located outside of individuals, and the other that culture is located inside people's minds. These two different orientations produce different implications as to how we treat the concept of culture.

Culture Outside Individuals

The first orientation—culture outside individuals—considers culture as a bounded whole, with which a group of people is defined and characterized. Individual differences are minimized at the expense of a coherent picture for the whole, and culture is seen to be observable and presentable as a public façade of a group. This view stems from the initial anthropological interest of studying other cultures by looking in from outside and is integrated into Kroeber and Kluckhohn's classic definition of culture originally published in 1952. The added italics accentuate this perspective of culture:

> Culture consists of patterns, explicit and implicit, of and for behavior, acquired and transmitted by symbols constituting the distinctive achievement of human groups, *including their embodiment in artifacts*; the essential core of culture consists of traditional (i.e., historically derived and selected) ideas and especially their attached values; *culture systems may, on the one hand, be considered as products of action, on the other as* conditioning elements of further action. (1966, p. 357)

This "looking-in-from-outside" perspective assumes that other cultures are observable. It creates the distance between anthropologists and local natives and, in turn, engenders the acute sense of difference and of clear boundaries between these two parties. As a result, anthropologists end up developing a sometimes essentialist and often exotic profile of culture to describe a bounded group of people, focusing on observable differences in custom, social structure, language, religion, art, and other material and nonmaterial characteristics. The oft-cited definition by Sir Edward Burnett Tylor (1871), who is characterized as "the founder of academic anthropology in the English-speaking world and the author of the first general anthropology textbook" (Harris, 1975, p. 144), also presents culture as a "complex whole" binding a group of people:

> Culture . . . taken in its wide ethnographic sense is that complex whole which includes knowledge, belief, art, morals, law, custom, and any other capabilities and habits acquired by man as a member of society. (Tylor, p. 1)

Tylor's definition illustrates the very point of this perspective, associating culture with an entire group of people.

De Munck (2000) identifies three versions of this culture-outside-individuals perspective: (1) "Culture is superorganic," (2) "Culture is public," and (3) "The size, position, and strength of social networks" affect the culture of a group (pp. 8–17). The first perspective, superorganic culture, still popular nowadays, postulates that a set group of people is identified with a culture and that culture has a life of its own, dictating, regulating, and controlling people to maintain inner-group "homogeneity." This perspective is illustrated by Benedict's two renowned works. In *Patterns of Culture* (1934) she classified cultures by two types—the orderly and calm "Apollonian" type and the emotional and passionate "Dionysian" type—and characterized Pueblo cultures of the American Southwest as the former and the Native American cultures of the Great Plains as the latter. Her notion of culture as a representation of a whole group also came through clearly in her discussion of Japanese "national culture" in *The Chrysanthemum and the Sword* (1946). My first student's notion of "American" culture is not far from this perspective of superorganic culture. So is Spring's notion of the U.S. "general" culture that is expected to consist of "behaviors, beliefs, and experiences common to most citizens" (2004, p. 4).

The second version of the culture-outside-individuals perspective is argued by Geertz, who sees culture forming in the process of people's interactive communication and meaning-making. Geertz (1973) holds that "culture is public because meaning is. . . . [C]ulture consists of socially established structures of meaning in terms of which people do such things as signal conspiracies and join them or perceive insults and answer them. . ." (pp. 12–13). For him, a person's behaviors cannot be appropriately understood and responded to unless these behaviors are publicly exhibited and others correctly interpret their meanings using the standards familiar to both parties.

The third version of the culture-outside-individuals perspective is apparent in Thompson's work, according to De Munck (2000). Thompson argues that "ensembles" of social relations, created by "social roles, statuses, and norms," affect the culture within a social organization (p. 12). This perspective postulates that culture is associated with the structure transcending individual distinctiveness. The "structure of any entity," including a society, refers to "the more-or-less enduring relationships among its parts" (Kaplan & Manners, 1972, p. 101) and "the continuing arrangement of persons in relationships defined or controlled by institutions" in Radcliffe-Brown's words (1958, p. 177). This social structure "contains" culture according to this view of culture outside individuals.

When this perspective of culture outside individuals swings to the extreme, it is in danger of presenting culture in a form of a lifeless, rigid mannequin—exaggerated, oversimplified, inflexible, and simply artificial—without reflecting real people associated with it or in a form of a self-propelled entity independent of people. In these cases the concept of culture intends to represent something, yet actually says little about people because it is so distanced from them.

Culture in People's Minds

In contrast to the first perspective, the second perspective locates culture in people's minds. In this case, human beings are regarded not only as bearers of culture but also as active agents who create, transmit, transform, and sometimes discard certain cultural traits. According to De Munck (2000), three versions constitute this perspective: (1) the "psychoanalytic and 'human nature' thesis of culture," (2) "personal and public symbols," and (3) cognitively distributed culture.

The first version is supported by Spiro, who rejects cultural determinism—the claim that a societal culture determines the personality of its members and shapes national personality. Instead, he argues that psychological similarities and differences between members of a culture also exist in other cultures. For him, "cultures are systems that function to meet the psychological and biological requirements of human beings as members of society" (De Munck, 2000, p. 19). Since basic human psychology and biology are similar as well as different from society to society, Spiro's observation that "the surface variations in cultures mask underlying similarities" puts this perspective in diametric opposition to the "superorganic culture" perspective that postulates distinctive cultural differences between groups. Erickson's classification of culture "as motive and emotion" is also aligned with this perspective of culture in that people's emotions and motives in their minds are driving forces in their social customs and actions (2004, p. 36).

De Munck (2000) associates Obeyesekere with the second version—"personal and public symbols." According to him, Obeyesekere vacillates "between asserting that culture is in or outside the body," like most contemporary psychoanalytical anthropologists (p. 19). In this version, culture is sometimes viewed as a passive set of ideas located inside meaning-makers and other times as an active agent organizing the society outside individuals. This version recognizes the complex dialectical relationship between culture and people. Erickson's classification of culture as "symbol system" is aligned with this view of culture in that culture is considered as "a more limited set of large chunks of knowledge . . . that frame or constitute what is taken as 'reality' by members of a social group" (2004, p. 36). The members use the knowledge to communicate with each other and regulate each other's behaviors. In this perspective, the knowledge (symbols) exists outside individuals until it is utilized by people; then it enters their minds.

The third version of the culture-in-people's-minds perspective is advocated strongly among cognitive anthropologists who assert that culture consists of cognitive schemas or standards that shape and define people's social experiences and interactions with others. Goodenough (1981) defines culture as "standards for perceiving, evaluating, believing, and doing" (p. 78). When individuals develop their versions of group culture, the individual versions become their "propriospects" in Goodenough's term and "idioverses" in Schwartz's (1978) term.

The view of culture inside people's mind helps people see themselves as active agents of culture. At the same time, when the role of individuals is excessively elevated in culture-making, this perspective is in danger of neglecting the collectivistic nature of "culture." When this happens, the division of psychology and anthropology is likely to be blurred.

A Work-in-Progress Concept of Culture

Acknowledging the potential shortcomings of both perspectives on the locus of culture, here I propose a work-in-progress concept of culture for this book, which is founded on seven premises.

Individuals are cultural agents, but culture is not at all about individuality. Culture is inherently collectivistic, not individualistic. Culture needs the individual "self" as well as others to exist. Therefore, the notion of "individual culture" connoting individual uniqueness defies the core of the concept of culture.

Individuals are not prisoners of culture. Rather, they exercise a certain level of autonomy when acquiring, transmitting, altering, creating, and shedding cultural traits while interacting with others. This individual autonomy is the foundation of inner-group diversity.

Despite inner-group diversity, a certain level of sharedness, common understanding, and/or repeated interactions is needed to bind people together as a group. A formal and official, even intentional, process is not always required to obtain membership of a cultural group. However, a degree of actual and imaginary connection with other members would be needed for them to become part of a collective culture and to claim an identity with the cultural group.

Individuals can become members of multiple social organizations concurrently. In Thompson's terms (1994), some organizations are "egocentric" (with micro-level structures where individuals are more intimately involved) and others "sociocentric" (with macro-level structures such as nations). Some memberships such as race or gender are more likely to be ascribed early in life and others can be achieved later by social or educational affiliations. So, one can be an American citizen, African American, female, graduate of Yale Law School, civil rights activist, and child advocate all at the same time, as in the case of Edelman (1999).

Each membership contributes to the cultural makeup of individuals with varying degrees of influence. Individuals develop varied levels of affinity and identity with different groups of people. The strength of affinity and identity with certain memberships fluctuates, depending on life circumstances. Agar (2006) illustrated this point well with his example of Catholic identity:

> I grew up in a parish with an old Irish priest, so we got that un- enlightened 1950s rural-Irish-gloom-and-doom-and-then-off- to-hell-you-go version. By high school, I thought of myself as an ex-Catholic. When I was about 30, I realized I'd never be ex. Nowadays, Mother Church is mostly a source of stories and jokes, except for the days when I feel like a defrocked Jesuit. The way that my religious culture comes and goes and fits or aggravates the flow of the moment changes from year to year, or even from moment to moment.

Other identities also vacillate, depending on the context in which people are placed. Some people have stronger ethnic identity than others; others have a stronger affinity with their primary groups than with nations. Over time, their primary identities—with the strongest sense of affinity—can shift as life circumstances change. For example, Crane's (2000) interview-based research revealed that during Nazi rule in Germany, female children of Christian-Jewish mixed marriages, who had been integrated into the mainstream German society, became much more cognizant of their Jewish roots and voluntarily and involuntarily took on a strong Jewish identity; this newly acquired identity ended up outliving the Nazi era.

Individuals can discard a membership of a cultural group with or without "shedding" their cultural traits. The effect of certain cultural memberships on people's day-to-day operation can be varied even long after they cease to associate intimately with members of cultural communities. For example, immigrants who change citizenship do not often abandon their native culture and language upon naturalization into their host country. The official abandonment of their original nationality may be refashioned in strict observation of certain cultural practices.

Without securing official memberships in certain cultural groups, obvious traits of membership, or members' approvals, outsiders can acquire cultural traits and claim cultural affiliations with other cultural groups. For example, Olson (1993), a self-ordained Christian missionary, went to Motilone Indian territory in Colombia and Venezuela, learned their language and customs, and became an advocate of the group to the outside world. Without an innate membership, he gained cultural and linguistic knowledge—"languaculture" in Agar's term (2006)—for access to people in the society, which eventually led him to an "affiliate" membership.

The Concepts of Self

Building on these seven premises of culture, I depart from cultural determinism (culture determines group personality) or cultural essentialism (identifiable cultural distinctiveness is relegated to a certain culture). Rather, I see culture as a product of interactions between self and others in a community of practice. In my thinking, an individual becomes a basic unit of culture. From this individual's point of view, self is the starting point for cultural acquisition and transmission. For this reason, scholars of culture pay a great deal of attention to the concept of self. Interestingly, the concept of self varies at different times and in different cultures.

Historical Concepts of Self

Interest in the concept of self has a long history in the Western scholarly tradition. From early Greek philosophers such as Socrates, to early Christian theologians such as St. Augustine (1999, Trans.), to contemporary postmodern scholars such as Gergen (1991), to contemporary psychologists such as Vitz (1977), the discussion of self has been rich and prolific. According to De Munck (2000), the term "self" was not always used in a positive light as it is in contemporary U.S. society. In its first appearance, around the 1300s, it was "used as a noun that packaged sin with the self" (p. 31). So, self was to be denied:

neither to be indulged nor celebrated, but rather to be shunned and ignored. Vitz's notion of "selfism" describes the undesired indulgence of self. This view of self has transformed over time.

Gergen (1991) surveys the changes in the concept of self from the romantic perspective of the 19th century, through the modern one of the 20th century, to the postmodern view of the contemporary era. He characterizes the 19th-century romantic view of self as "one that attributes to each person characteristics of personal depth: passion, soul, creativity, and moral fiber" (p. 6). From this perspective, a person's emotion, feeling, and intuition are considered integral to selfhood. In contrast to the romantic view, modernists deemphasize the affective and intuitive attributes of self and highlight the characteristics of the self residing "in our ability to reason—in our beliefs, opinions, and conscious intentions" (p. 6). With the scientific advances of the 20th century, a person's reason and objectivity are far more valued. However, contemporary postmodernists are skeptics of this modernist sense of a rational, orderly self. Gergen claims, "Selves as possessors of real and identifiable characteristics—such as rationality, emotion, inspiration, and will—are dismantled" in the postmodern view (p. 7). The modern belief in "moral imperatives" and autonomous self (Grenz, 1996; Taylor, 1989) is replaced by the postmodernists' recognition of a "saturated" self that is overcommitted to often divergent pulling forces and demands of surroundings, and a "protean self," in Lifton's term, that constantly adjusts to "turbulent, dislocating, and often violent global forces and conditions" (De Munck, 2000, p. 44).

Although the postmodern view of self might have deprived us of a hope for a self-sufficient, independent, and directional self, it invites us to look at self as a "fragile" and interdependent being. Gergen (1991) articulates the reality of interdependency thus: "[O]ne's sense of individual autonomy gives way to a reality of immersed interdependence, in which it is relationship that constructs the self" (p. 147). The attention to community is another contribution of postmodernism to the scholarship of self: "the continued existence of humankind is dependent on a new attitude of cooperation rather than conquest" vis-à-vis community (p. 7). The recognition of self in relation to community is one of the four insights we could gain from the postmodern perspective according to Hjorkbergen (cited in Meneses, 2000).

The postmodern recognition that human beings are not truly independent and autonomous is ironically aligned with the Christian assessment of humanity. While some Christian scholars criticize the postmodern notion of the directionless self lost in moral relativism, they may easily embrace the notion of the fragile self in need of relationships with the Creator and other human beings. As Apostle Paul reminds us, "so in Christ [the incarnated Creator] we who are many form one body, and each member belongs to all the other" (Romans 12:5, New International Version). Although Christianity has provided a foundation for Western thought, its notion of self is different from the Western modern secular view of the self-confident, self-reliant, and independent self. Rather, the Christian self, before and after St. Augustine, does not deny its reliance upon others, whether God or other human beings.

Cross-Cultural Concepts of Self

The concept of self has evolved not only historically but also is cross-culturally varied. Gergen's discussion of the romantic, modern, and postmodern self draws upon the Western secular view of self as "a bounded, unique, more or less integrated motivational and cognitive universe, a dynamic center of awareness, emotion, judgment, and action. . ." (Geertz, 1984, p. 126). Geertz warns that such a view of self is "a rather peculiar idea within the context of the world's culture." Thus it is entirely possible to view self as something other than a unique, separate, and autonomous being to be distinguished from others and to be elevated as the center of the universe above a community. Comparing the Western view of self with that of the Wintu (Lee, 1959) and the Oglala (Lee, 1986), Lee acknowledges that the sense of self in these Native Americans does not rest on the contradiction between self and other; instead, self and other are viewed as mutually inclusive. For Oglala, "the self contains some of the other, participates in the other, and is in part contained within the other. . . . [I]n respecting the other, the self is simultaneously respected" (1986, p. 12). Hoffman (1996) also criticizes the fact that "individual uniqueness" is overemphasized as the tenet of self in the Western scholarship of multicultural education because in many non-Western cultural contexts celebration of the individual self is not always valued and self does not always take precedence over others in the decision-making process.

Collectivism,[1] illustrated in the aforementioned Native American cultures, is not always a non-Western ethos. Valuing a community over individuals was apparent in the first-century Mediterranean culture that permeates the New Testament writings. Malina (1993) uses the term "dyadism," in lieu of "collectivism," to describe the "strong group orientation," manifested in the New Testament culture, in which "persons always considered themselves as inextricably embedded . . . conceive[d] of themselves as always interrelated with other persons while occupying a distinct social position both horizontally . . . and vertically" and "live[d] out the expectations of others" (p. 67). In such a culture, selfhood is understood only in relation to others within a community.

Autoethnography benefits greatly from the thought that self is an extension of a community rather than that it is an independent, self-sufficient being, because the possibility of cultural self-analysis rests on an understanding that self is part of a cultural community.

The Concepts of Others

The recognition of varying dynamics between self and others allows us to segue into a discussion of "others." The scholarly interest in "othering" has increased in the society of cultural diversity (Asher, 2001; Canales, 2000; Luke, 1994). Human beings have always developed mental and social mechanisms to differentiate "us" from "them." In the process, they develop criteria for others.

The Typology of Others

The term "others" generally refers to existentially different human beings—those who are other than self. The differences that separate self from others "often shift with time, distance, and perspective" (Canales, 2000, p. 16). Not all existential others pose the same level of strangeness to self. Those who belong to the same community as self are likely to be seen as comrades who share similar standards and values. These are *others of similarity.* On the other hand, others from a different community are likely to be distinguished as strangers who possess and operate by different frames of reference. In identifying others of difference, the perception of difference may play just as powerful a role as actual differences. When differences in behaviors, beliefs, or customs are deemed to be not only irreconcilable but also threatening to the very existence of self and others of similarity, the others are regarded as *others of opposition*, namely "enemies" to their neighborhood, interest group, school, professional organization, or nation. The typology of others—of similarity, difference, and opposition—is helpful in understanding self and its interconnectedness with others, especially as a framework for the autoethnographic data analysis and interpretation that will be discussed in Chapter 9.

Cultural Verstehen of Others

I have already postulated that culture is intertwined with people. This implies that cultural understanding of others begins with genuine encounters with them through which insider perspectives are gained. A genuine relationship develops from an "I–Thou" encounter, as opposed to an "I–It" encounter, according to Martin Buber (Panko, 1976). In this I–Thou encounter, people acknowledge human dignity in each other (Pohl, 1999) and are engaged in genuine dialogue "as a person to a person, as a subject to a subject" (Panko, p. 48). The opposite of the I–Thou interaction is the I–It encounter in which one treats others as objects. Buber does not deny the value of the I–It encounter as a realm in which "we are able to examine all things critically and verify or disapprove what we have experienced" (p. 54), yet he acknowledges that the I–Thou encounter is the only realm where those engaged in dialogue can experience each other's whole being. Neither pretense nor insincerity has a place in this relationship.

In addition to genuine encounters, a true understanding of others also requires empathic understanding—"verstehen," in German sociologist-philosopher Max Weber's term. Empathic understanding is an act of putting aside one's own framework and "seeing [others'] experiences within the framework of their own" (Geertz, 1984, p. 126). Although perfect verstehen is beyond our human capacity, attempts to empathize can reduce incorrect judgments about others and enhance rich understanding of strangers. This empathic understanding is, in a Malinowskian–Geertzian sense, understanding "from the native's point of view," on which a rich contextual understanding of others' culture is grounded. These steps of understanding are equally helpful in understanding others of both similarity and difference.

Yet understanding others of similarity and difference requires a different course of action on the part of self. To continue the discussion we need to revisit the concept of self as a relational being. This concept of self presupposes the existence of relational partners. In other words, self cannot exist alone in the context of culture. Others from the primary community (e.g., family or religious community) and the secondary community (e.g., professional or interest organization) participate in the production of self in the enculturation or socialization process.[2] Self learns values, norms, and customs from others to become a proper member of the community. Self contributes to the continuity of the community as well. In this give-and-take process, self is invariably bound with others within the cultural group. Consequently, self becomes mirrored in others, and others become an extension of self.

Cultural presuppositions shared by self and others are the foundation of homogeneity, unity, and congruity within the community. In a culturally "congruent"[3] society, relating to others may not be such a daunting task. Others are merely others of similarity; thus, understanding others may easily begin with knowing and affirming self.

When "others" refers to members of other communities—others of difference—self and others are not organically interconnected; rather, such interconnectivity must be intentionally desired and achieved. In a diverse society composed of others from different ethnic, racial, religious, gender-orientation, ability, age, socioeconomic status, profession, civic orientation, or interest groups, relating to and understanding others requires a different course of action from merely affirming self as in a relatively homogeneous cultural context. Self may need to start with "denying self" by putting aside its own standards, crossing its own cultural boundaries, and "immersing" self in others' cultures (Lingenfelder, 1996). Totally breaking away from one's own culture is almost impossible and not desirable when attempting to achieve a healthy balance between affirming self and learning from others. Yet, leaving one's standards momentarily and observing and analyzing differences between self and others from a distance are helpful practices in understanding others of difference. In the process, self may learn from others and take in a part of others. The genuine effort to "*verstehen*" others' culture often engenders cultural crossing between self and others.

Expanding Cultural Boundaries

The product of genuine and thoughtful cultural crossing is known as an "edgewalker" according to Kreb (1999). Edgewalkers have significant "lived" experiences with different cultural communities through which they develop solid cross-cultural competence while maintaining a healthy understanding of self. They exhibit the following qualities:

> 1) comfort, if not identification, with a particular ethnic, spiritual or cultural group, 2) competence thriving in mainstream culture, 3) the capacity to move between cultures in a way that an individual can discuss with some clarity, 4) the ability to generalize from personal experience to that of people from other groups without being trapped in the uniqueness of a particular culture. . . . (p. 1)

Blending old and new cultural competence, edgewalkers constantly turn their former others of difference into others of similarity by reducing strangeness in others and expanding their cultural boundaries. They also engage others in the mutually transformational process because genuine cross-cultural pollination affects both parties. As a result, both self and others end up expanding their cultural boundaries to include each other.

The notion of cross-cultural expansion can be applied at the societal level. Through genuine dialogues with others, a community can also expand its boundaries to include others of difference. Greene (2000) refers to such an inclusive community as an "extended community." This community is characterized as "attentive to difference, open to the idea of plurality" (p. 44), and grounded on "the desire to extend the reference of 'us' as far as we can" (p. 45). The extended community redefines the division of "us and them" and expands the boundaries to treat former others of difference as new others of similarity. In this case the notion of community is no longer founded on mere common characteristics among members, but on the shared ideology of democracy and inclusive wills (Thayer-Bacon & Bacon, 1998).

Summary

So far I have introduced three interconnecting concepts: culture, self, and others. The concept of culture, inherently group-oriented, was examined from two perspectives: culture outside individuals and culture in people's minds. Self, as a basic unit of culture, was also discussed from historical and cross-cultural perspectives. Although self has been viewed differently in different time periods and cultures, I argue that self is consistently connected to others in the realm of culture. The others refer to other human beings differently regarded by self: some are seen as others of similarity (friends to self), as others of difference (strangers to self), or as others of opposition (enemies to self). The view of others is not fixed in people's lives. Rather, the positionality of self to others is socially constructed and transformable as the self develops its relationship to others—especially strangers and enemies—and reframes its views of others. Understanding the relationship between self and others is one of the tasks that auto-ethnographers may undertake. In this sense, these three concepts are vital building blocks to the discussion of autoethnography, the primary focus of this book.

Self-Narratives

Telling stories is an ancient practice, perhaps as old as human history. Imagine a family clan sitting around a fire pit on a starry night to listen to the family's migration history. Or picture a grandmother rocking in a chair with her grandchildren on her lap, telling her childhood memories. As in these cases, stories can easily contain the autobiographical components of storytellers, even when the stories feature the storytellers' ancestors, families, relatives, neighbors, or communities. This autobiographical storytelling, also called self-narration, sometimes produces written narratives. Self-narratives, "personal narratives" in Gornick's (2001) term, refer to stories "written by people who, in essence, are imagining only themselves: in relation to the subject in hand" (p. 6).

Writings focusing on self have increased significantly in volume in recent decades, representing various genres, authorship, thematic focus, and writing styles. They have come in the form of autobiography, memoir, journal, diary, personal essay, or letter. Some organize autobiographical facts in chronological fashion; others assemble authors' personal reflections around various themes. Some use a more descriptive mode of storytelling like memoirs; yet others use autobiographical facts in "scholarly personal narratives" (Nash, 2004) or in autoethnography (Reed-Danahay, 1997), which tend to be more analytical and interpretive. In this chapter, I first discuss the value of self-narratives in cultural understanding of self and others and later expound on the variety of self-narratives with selected examples.

Growing Interest in Self-Narratives

Gornick (2001) notes the increasing popularity of self-narrative writing: "Thirty years ago people who thought they had a story to tell sat down to write a novel. Today they sit down to write a memoir" (p. 89). A search of the Library of Congress catalogs for the keywords of autobiography and memoir turned up 10,000 entries for each keyword. Lavery (1999) also compiled an extensive list of autobiographies. The growing popularity of contemporary self-narratives rides on the back of postmodernism that values voices of common people, defying the conventional authoritative elitism of autobiography (Wall, 2006). Ordinary authors with no political clout or literary credentials have gained courage to speak their stories.

Recently I came upon a memoir by Plourde (2005) prominently displayed in a university bookstore. Currently a university student, the author accounts her life-changing encounter with a cruel rape by a stranger, subsequent pregnancy, and a dilemma of deciding between abortion and pregnancy as a pro-lifer during her high school days. Obviously such a self-writing is publishable and readily available to readers.

The explosion of self-narratives has enriched the study of this type of writing but makes it an intimidating task to select examples to share because for every selected item many more are left unmentioned. An exhaustive literature review of self-narratives is beyond the scope of this chapter. With help of my graduate assistant Judy Ha, I have made a modest attempt to select and classify over 70 book-length self-narratives and anthologies into seven categories: (1) autoethnographies; (2) memoirs and autobiographies (MA)—racial, ethnic, and language issues; (3) MA—gender issues; (4) MA—religious issues; (5) MA—politics, social conflicts, and wars; (6) MA—childhood memories, family relations, and growing up; and (7) MA—disability, illness, and death. Appendix A presents a bibliography of self-narratives. In this chapter I simply share some examples of this vast genre.

An interest in studying self-narratives, as part of a broader trend of "narrative inquiry," has grown both in humanities and social sciences (Clandinin & Connelly, 2000; Ellis & Bochner, 2000). Memoir writing by literary writers has long dominated the scene of self-narratives in the humanities (Allende, 2003; Angelou, 1969; Baker, 1982;

Baldwin, 1963; De Beauvoir, 2005; Dillard, 1987; Hurston, 1984; Lamott, 2000 & 2005; Momaday, 1976; Rodriguez, 1982). Notable is social scientists' growing interest in self as a subject of academic inquiry (Burnier, 2006). The widespread interest in self-narratives has been demonstrated by scholars in anthropology (Anderson, 2000; Angrosino, 2007; Bateson, 1994 & 1995; Mead, 1972; Reed-Danahay, 1997), sociology (Denzin, 1997; Lucal, 1999; Richardson, 1992), communication (Ellis, 1995; Ellis & Bochner, 1996 & 2000), education (Florio-Ruane, 2001; Gallas, 1998; Obidah & Teel, 2001; Romo, 2004), medicine (Kübler-Ross & Gold, 1997), nursing (Foster, McAllister, & O'Brien, 2005), psychiatry (Jamison, 1996), and psychology (Schafer, 1992).

Ellis and Bochner (2000) note that social scientists' interest in self-narratives falls in one of the four categories: (1) "reflexive ethnographies" in which "authors use their own experiences in the culture reflexively to bend back on self and look more deeply at self–other interaction"; (2) "texts by complete-member researchers" who "explore groups of which they already are members or in which . . . they have become full members with complete identification and acceptance"; (3) "personal narratives" written by social scientists about "some aspect of their experience in daily life"; and (4) "literary autoethnography" written by an autobiographical writer who "focuses as much on examining self autobiographically as on interpreting a culture for a nonnative audience" (p. 740). The common theme underlying all these diverse labels is self-focus.

Although self-narratives focus on the author, self-stories often contain more than self. The irony of self-narratives is that they are of self but not self alone. Others often enter self-narratives as persons intimately and remotely connected to self. As a relational being, the self is invariably connected to others in the family, local and national community, and world, "a series of overlapping, concentric circles with others" in Nash's (2002, p. 26) terms. Friends, acquaintances, and even strangers from the circles are interwoven in self-narratives. Therefore, studying and writing of self-narratives is an extremely valuable activity in understanding self and others connected to self.

Self-Narratives for Understanding Self and Others

Reading and studying others' self-narratives is hardly a one-sided activity that results only in understanding others. Studying others invariably invites readers to compare and contrast themselves with others in the cultural texts they read and study, in turn discovering new dimensions of their own lives.

Florio-Ruane (2001) observed the value of using autobiographies, specifically written by writers of color, in her graduate multicultural education course. She argues that reading these self-narratives for discussion helped her education students, predominantly White middle-class females, learn about different cultures presented by the autobiographers of Asian, Hispanic, African American, and Native American cultural backgrounds while they examined their own cultural assumptions through self-reflection.

Expanding from reading self-narratives, Brunner (1994) advocates inservice teachers' utilizing a variety of texts—not only books but also film or television scripts and musical lyrics—created by others to evoke self-reflection and self-analysis. She argues, "As students are called on to explore their own personal histories, their social, political, economic, and cultural realities through a curriculum of multiple voices, their predispositions tend to become more apparent" (p. 235). For both Florio-Ruane (2001) and Brunner (1994), self-reflection evoked by reading of others is a means to self-discovery.

Self-discovery in a cultural sense is intimately related to understanding others. If "others" refers to members of one's own community (others of similarity), the self is reflected in others in a general sense. Values and standards upheld by the community are likely shared between self and others. Although people do not practice the values and standards of their community in minute detail, the knowledge of the values and standards helps them understand others of similarity from their own community. Therefore, understanding others could smooth the transition to understanding self. If "others" refers to members of other communities (others of difference), understanding the similarity between self and others captures only a portion of understanding others. What is beneficial in this case is studying others thoroughly through comparing and contrasting, which inevitably brings differences to light.

Studying others has a value in itself. However, Hall (1973) and Noel (2000) consider that it has a greater purpose of helping to understand self. Hall unapologetically argues that "the real job" of studying another culture is "not to understand foreign culture but to understand our own . . . to learn more about how one's own system works" (p. 30). Noel chimes in: "the study of [other] culture is the study of our own lives, of our own ways of thinking and living" (p. 81). Whether seeing self through others or against others, the study of self-narratives through self-reflection is beneficial to cultural understanding.

The Variety of Self-Narratives

"Self-narratives" cover a wide range of writings whose primary focus rests on self. Besides the commonality, they vary in genre, authorship, thematic focus, and writing style. Although the purpose of this chapter is not to provide a full-scale literature review of self-narratives, the variety of self-narratives will be discussed here to provide a context for the discussion of autoethnography that follows in the next chapter.

Genres

All writings are in some ways autobiographical because they reflect authors' perspectives and preferences in their choices of topic, writing style, direction, and conclusion. However, in this genre study of self-narratives, I will discuss only writings that demonstrate an author's explicit intention of bringing self to the surface as an object of description, analysis, and/or interpretation.

With the intentionality of self-exposure in mind, scholars of self-narratives consider St. Augustine's *Confessions* (1999) from the 4th century CE as "something of a model for the memoirist," in which "Augustine tells the tale of his conversion to Christianity" (Gornick, 2001, p. 13). This tradition of confession continued in the spiritual account of a 15th-century English mystic Margery Kempe (2000); spiritual journals of 17th-century Puritan New Englanders such as Sarah Osborn, Susanna Anthony, Harriett Newell, Fanny Woodbury, and Abigail Bailey (Taves, 1992); and Daniel Shea (Mason, 1992). Contemporary spiritual self-narratives in the United States are not limited to Protestantism (Carter, 1996; Lamott, 2000, 2005; Lewis, 1956; Olson, 1993) or Catholicism (Armstrong, 2005; Breyer, 2000; Crossan, 2000; Donofrio, 2000; Hathaway, 1992; Merton, 1999; Norris, 1996), but embrace other faiths or spiritual traditions such as Islam (Ahmedi & Ansary, 2005), Zen Buddhism (Brooks, 2000; Goldberg, 1993), Judaism (Dubner, 1999), and feminine spirituality (Kidd, 2002).

The tradition of self-accounts did not stop in the religious realm. Self-narratives have been broadly adopted in contemporary secular literature in the form of autobiography, memoir, journal, personal essay, and letter. Autobiography is probably the most well-known format of self-narratives. Autobiography tends, chronologically and comprehensively, to depict lives of authors, who are often distinguished as public figures such as the first female Secretary of State, Madeleine Albright (2003), U.S. President Jimmy Carter (1996), U.S.

President Bill Clinton (2004), First Lady Hillary Rodham Clinton (2004), abolitionist and suffragist Frederick Douglass (1995), Indian political activist Mahatma Gandhi (1957), South African President Nelson Mandela (1994), civil rights activist Rosa Parks (1992), First Lady Eleanor Roosevelt (1984), and civil rights activist Malcolm X (Haley & Malcolm X, 1996). The social importance of autobiographers often adds formality to this genre of self-narratives.

Memoir has become a more common option for contemporary writers because this format allows a thematic approach to one's life story but with moderation in scope. Memoirs tend to focus on fragments of memoirists' lives, not the whole life. Phifer (2002) differentiates memoirs from autobiographies in terms of the focus of time:

> Autobiographies present broad overviews, while memoirs focus on only the hours and minutes that are keen in our lives—the times when we are most alive, when experiences penetrate to the quick. In these moments we define ourselves; the ways we respond reveal our souls. (p. 4)

Memoirs tend to follow themes around which memoirists gather autobiographical stories. For example, Ann Lamott's *Traveling Mercies* (2000) focuses on the author's spiritual conversion and development; and Jane Tompkins (1996) narrates the story of her involvement in education as a student and later as a professor in *A Life in School*.

Memoirs are also different from journals. According to Phifer (2002), memoirs are more "selective," with a focus on "the most significant experiences in their lives and then [organizing] their chapters in a sequence that tells a story," while journals "tend to be logs or records of daily growth, musings, and insights" and may feel more "fragmentary" than memoirs (p. 4). Nevertheless, journal writing commonly engages in self-reflection and self-description. Similarly, diaries are used to record daily happenings; they tend to be more chronological and descriptive of the happenings. Both journals and diaries are usually written for the authors themselves, although some end up being published for broader audiences. These formats are valuable to self-narratives because the content often reveals less self-censored behavior and thought. Anthropologists' field journals, and travel journals, war diaries, and spiritual journals, to name a few, exemplify this genre. Anderson's (2000) reflections on her fieldworks and Malinowski's (1967) field diary fall in this category.

The personal essay is another genre of self-narrative. It does not chronicle an author's life per se. It contains personal insights in response to the author's environment. Gornick (2001) argues that a personal essay combines "personal journalism . . . [and] social criticism" and should fall into "the pit of confessionalism or therapy on the page or naked self-absorption" (p. 9). Nevertheless, personal essays have a potential to be self-narratives when they fully expose the authors' perspectives. Letters can also have self-narrative quality when they contain descriptions of the behaviors and thoughts of their authors. Abigail Adams's letters to her husband, John Adams, during the Revolutionary War also became famous as documents revealing her political thoughts on roles of women (Sinopoli, 1997).

Despite the differences in formality, scope, and format, all genres of self-narrative share the common activities of memory search, self-revelation through personal stories, and self-reflection in the process.

Authorship

Conventionally, socially distinguished individuals were considered worthy authors for autobiography or memoir. However, the authorship of self-narratives has become noticeably diversified during the last three decades, to include more historically underrepresented populations, such as people of color (Angelou, 1969), women (Halverson, 2004; McKay, 1998; Sands, 1992), gays and lesbians (Bepko, 1997), and people with disabilities (Fries, 1997).

Self-narratives are generally penned by the "owners" of stories. That is to say, storytellers are identical to authors. In some cases, however, narrators tell their stories to writers who transcribe and edit the stories to varying degrees. Although the narrators still ensure the authority of the stories, the writers are often nevertheless credited. Narrative of Sojourner Truth (Gilbert with Sojourner Truth, 1997), The Autobiography of Malcolm X (Haley with Malcolm X, 1996), and Sun Chief: The Autobiography of a Hopi Indian (edited by Simmons, 1942) are products of such collaboration between socially distinguished figures and professional writers. North American slave narratives took a similar course of documentation when writers and journalists between 1936 and 1938 interviewed over 2,300 former slaves from across the American South to record their lives as slaves. Although most slave narrators have not been elevated to the status of the aforementioned authors, the process of self-narration and documentation was similar.

Thematic Focus

Self-narratives can also be varied depending on the themes they adopt. Themes adopted by self-narrators are as diverse as the authorship is widespread. In this section, I provide just a few examples so that readers may gain the sense of open-endedness in the thematic focus of self-narratives. Some examples include education (Adams, 2007), professorship (Nash, 2002), politics (Albright, 2003), biraciality (Lazarre, 1996; McBride, 1996; Walker, 2001), Mexican-American ethnicity (Rodriguez, 1982; Romo, 2004), religion (Olson, 1993), sexual orientation (Bepko, 1997), disability (Dubus, 1998), love, AIDS, and death of a husband (Peterson, 2003), father-son relationship (Ackerley, 1975; Lott, 1997), and mother-daughter relationship (Corse, 2004).

The thematic focus of some self-narratives is singular in that the entire writing centers on one theme. Richard Rodriguez' (1982) memoir, *Hunger of Memory*, illustrates a singular themed self-narrative in which he describes his assimilating educational experience growing up as a son of a Mexican immigrant in California. His singular focus is contrasted with the multi-faceted memoir of Colin Powell (with Persico, 1995), another child of an immigrant from Jamaica. However, Powell's memoir addresses many other aspects of his life, from education and family to military and political career.

One thematic focus that may interest educators is teaching. As self-reflection for educational practitioners is strongly advocated in teacher education, more educators are engaging in self-reflective narration in the form of cultural autobiography (Chang, 1999; Kennett, 1999) and teacher autobiography (Brookfield, 1995; Clausen & Cruickshank, 1991; Nieto, 2003; Powell, Zehm, & Garcia, 1996; Tiedt & Tiedt, 2005). Others have engaged in teacher research in which they self-observe their teaching practices, examine their relationship with students, and reflect on their teaching philosophy. Obidah and Teel (2001) discuss their professional and Black-White cross-racial relationship as teaching colleagues in a mentoring relationship; Gallas (1998) analyzes her observation of and response to the relationship between boys and girls in her elementary classroom. These teacher research pieces reveal not only the authors' teaching practices but also the cultural assumptions they bring to self-examination. As teachers face increasing cultural diversity in the classroom, their interest in using self-narratives as cultural texts to analyze themselves and others will only grow.

Writing Styles

Self-narratives employ various writing styles such as descriptive/self-affirmative, analytical/interpretive, and confessional/self-critical/self-evaluative. Although different styles may be mixed in a particular self-narrative, one particular style of writing may be pronounced in a narrative depending on the intent of the narrator. The descriptive style of writing tends to be prominent in literary memoirs, in which stories themselves are of high value. An excerpt from Maya Angelou's (1969) first volume of autobiography, *I Know Why the Caged Bird Sings,* illustrates descriptive/self-affirmative writing. She describes her grandmother ("Momma"), one of the most important figures in her early development, who led her to become a confident African American woman:

> We lived with our grandmother and uncle in the rear of the Store (it was always spoken of with a capitals), which she had owned some twenty-five years.
>
> Early in the century, Momma (we soon stopped calling her Grand-mother) sold lunches to the sawmen in the lumberyard (east Stamps) and the seedmen at the cotton gin (west Stamps). Her crisp meat pies and cool lemonade, when joined to her miraculous ability to be in two places at the same time, assured her business success. From being a mobile lunch counter, she set up a stand between the two points of fiscal interest and supplied the workers' needs for a few years. Then she had the Store built in the heart of the Negro area. Over the years it became the lay center of activities in town. On Saturdays, barbers sat their customers in the shade on the porch of the Store, and troubadours on their ceaseless crawlings through the South leaned across its benches and sang their sad songs of The Brazos while they played juice harps and cigar-box guitars. (p. 7)

Her grandmother is here depicted as a smart businesswoman who glued the local African American community together. Acknowledgment of her grandmother's strength, intelligence, and caring simultaneously affirms where the narrator came from and who she is. Through stories like this, Angelou also affirms the inherent value of her own life experiences as an African American woman.

Differing from this descriptive writing style, an analytical and interpretive style tends to dominate anthropological and sociological scholarly writings in which autobiographical stories are treated as materials to analyze rather than as a centerpiece to appreciate. Azoulay's (1997) personal story of Black-Jewish interracial heritage is adopted for such a purpose.

> I was born and raised in the United States and am of Jewish and West Indian descent. As a child, my mother escaped Nazi Austria, where Jews were listed as a *racial* category. My father emigrated to the United States as a young boy. His ancestral genealogy includes ancestors from Cuba and Scotland and relatives, by marriage, of Chinese descent. My 1952 New York City birth certificate classified my father's "Race" as "Negro" and my mother as "White," thus designating me a Negro—by law. I lived in Israel for twenty-one years, and my Israel identity card registers only my "Nationality," as Jewish. This background informs my perspective, influences my opinions, and shapes the manner in which I have engaged with the people I have interviewed. (p. 19)

As it is written, it may appear quite similar to Angelou's descriptive writing. However, the reader would soon find out that this personal story serves only as a thematic anchor for Azoulay's book, *Black, Jewish, and Interracial*. She offers no other personal stories of significance besides this description of her racial identity. This story provides an entry point to many stories of other Black-Jewish interracials. She analyzes and interprets in an autoethnographic manner the stories of others who share the same racial identity with her. This approach to her personal story allows her to keep a distance from her own and others' similar stories to analyze and interpret the racial discourse of the United States.

Confessional/self-critical/self-evaluative writing tends to expose self—inequities, problems, or troubles—providing a vehicle through which self-narrators work to come to resolution or self-learning. Spiritual memoirs, personal journals, and diaries may be friendly to this type of writing. Lamott's narration of her imperfect past, an encounter with God's grace, conversion from atheism to faith, and transformation in her relationship with others illustrates this writing style. The following excerpt describes her conversion experience after her long downward-spiral experiences with alcoholism, drug abuse, heavy smoking, and abortion:

> And I was appalled. I thought about my life and my brilliant hilarious progressive friends, I thought about what everyone would think of me if I became a Christian, and it seemed an utterly

impossible thing that simply could not be allowed to happen. I turned to the wall and said out loud, "I would rather die."

I felt him just sitting there on his haunches in the corner of my sleeping loft, watching me with patience and love and I squinted my eyes shut, but that didn't help because that's not what I was seeing him with. . . . And one week later, when I went back to church, I was so hungover that I couldn't stand up for the songs, and this time I stayed for the sermon. . . . I began to cry and left before the benediction, and I raced home and felt the little cat running along at my heels. . . . I opened the door to my houseboat, and I stood there a minute, and then I hung my head and said, ". . . I quit." I took a long deep breath and said out loud, "All right, you can come in."

So this was my beautiful moment of conversion. (pp. 49–50)

Classifying the multitude of self-narratives by these three writing styles is challenging because an entire self-narrative is rarely fixed by one writing style. By understanding the typology of writing styles, however, self-narrators will be able to match writing styles with writing purposes.

Summary

Self-narratives refer to a wide range of written accounts of self, representing diverse genres, authorship, themes, and writing styles. They not only record personal stories of self-narrators but also embrace the sociocultural contexts of the stories. Therefore, writing one's own self-narratives and studying other self-narratives are valuable in learning about self and others, particularly in a cultural sense. The writing process evokes self-reflection and self-analysis through which self-discovery becomes a possibility. The study of other self-narratives helps readers compare and contrast their lives with those of self-narrators. This cognitive activity of compare and contrast engenders self-examination and self-learning. The variety of self-narratives only attests to their increased recognition in humanities and social sciences. In the next chapter I provide an in-depth discussion of autoethnography, a form of self-narrative adopted in the social sciences.

Autoethnography

In the previous chapter, I discussed the waxing interest in self-narratives in the contemporary scholarship of the humanities and social sciences. Here I single out autoethnography from the complex landscape of self-narratives to discuss its distinctive characteristics and application in the social sciences. Stemming from the field of anthropology, autoethnography shares the storytelling feature with other genres of self-narrative but transcends mere narration of self to engage in cultural analysis and interpretation. It is this analytical and interpretive nature that I focus on in distinguishing autoethnography from other self-narratives. Following a general discussion in this chapter of autoethnography's history, characteristics, benefits, and the pitfalls to avoid, methodological specifics are presented in Part II.

Autoethnography, Anthropology, and Social Sciences

Attention to self and autobiographical narratives is not new to social scientists, including anthropologists (Anderson, 2006; Atkinson, 2006; Best, 2006; Burnier, 2006; Denzin, 2006; Denzin & Lincoln, 2000). Whether they believe culture to be located "out there, in the public world" or "in here, in the private sphere of the self," none of the scholars refutes the basic premise that culture and individuals are intricately intertwined. Particularly, anthropologists who locate culture "in the private sphere of the self" value individual interpretations of culture without abandoning the very basic notion of group orientation of culture shared by group members. Goodenough's (1981) notion of "propriospect," developed further by Wolcott (1991), refers to an individual version of culture and illustrates this school of thinking. Namely, this concept implies that the basic unit of culture is individuals who can actively interpret their social surroundings.

Anthropological interest in individuals has traditionally manifested itself in life histories, mostly involving self-narratives of informants. Life histories such as *Sun Chief* (Simmons, 1942) are typical in that an informant's life is the focal point of study. In the case of *Sun Chief*, a Hopi Indian Chief told his life history to the anthropologist-author who wrote down the stories and added his anthropological interpretation. Some anthropologists have explored life histories of their own family members. This type of life history is exemplified by *Through Harsh Winters* (Kikumura, 1981), in which the author studied her mother who emigrated from Japan at the turn of the century. Brettell (1997) also combines the elements of biography and autobiography in the autoethnographical study of her mother who was a successful journalist. In both works, the researchers' autobiographies are invariably enmeshed with their mothers' biographies.

Another form of autobiographical involvement in self comes in the category of "native ethnographies," ethnographies conducted by ethnographers about their own people. Brayboy's (2005) study of Native American graduate students in an Ivy League university falls in this category because of his personal background similar to his informants'. As ethnographers turn their attention to home and traditionally studied groups produce their own anthropologists, native ethnographies are on the rise.

The third type of autobiographical writings involves anthropologists more intimately. "Confessional tales" (Van Maanen, 1988), "ethnographic memoirs" (Ellis & Bochner, 2000), and "reflexive ethnographies" (Tedlock, 2000) fall in this category in which ethnographers expose their ethnographic process, their personal experiences, or feelings from the field. Malinowski's field "diary" (1967) is considered one of the first ethnographic memoirs that describe "what went on in the backstage of doing research" (Ellis & Bochner, 2000, p. 741). In a similar fashion, Spindler (1983) compiled fieldwork experiences by 11 anthropologists in his edited book, and Anderson (2000) reflects on her anthropological fieldwork in 10 countries in the course of 30 years.

Anthropologists have also been engaged in memoir writing. Mead's (1972) *Blackberry Winter* and her daughter Bateson's (1994) *With a Daughter's Eye* exemplify this self-narrative of a sort. Margeret Mead's memoir describes her childhood and her adulthood as an anthropologist; Bateson reveals the lives of two legendary anthropologists, Margaret Mead and Gregory Bateson, from the perspective of their only daughter. These writings primarily focus on their lives, not their ethnographic work. Yet, their cultural insights permeate their memoirs.

Acknowledging the long-standing interest of anthropologists in self, Reed-Danahay (1997) states, "We are in the midst of renewed interest in personal narrative, in life history, and in autobiography among anthropologists" (p. 1). By the "renewed interest in self-narrative," however, Reed-Danahay alludes to something more than the four categories of anthropological scholarship of self mentioned above. It certainly transcends the traditional anthropological interest in other perspectives on "self" (Lee, 1986) or the inevitable insertion of the ethnographer self in his/her ethnographic work, as Goldschmidt (1977) articulated in his presidential address at the 1976 American Anthropological Association meeting: "In a sense, all ethnography is self-ethnography" (p. 294). The "new" trend of self-focused anthropology is based on intentional self-reflexivity; anthropologists are turning their scholarly interest inward on themselves. By articulating and reviving the term autoethnography, Reed-Danahay (1997) not only reminds us of anthropologists' long-standing interest in self, but also liberates a new generation of anthropologists to bring their personal stories to the center stage of their investigation.

Despite the long-standing interest in self in anthropology, self-reflexivity has not been readily embraced by some anthropologists and social scientists. Salzman (2002) is one of the critics of reflexivity. He argues that the postmodern obsession with self-reflexivity and with ethnographer subjectivity stalls the progress of anthropology. His critique illustrates the existing tug of war between two positions—objectivity vs. subjectivity—in social science. The objectivity position promotes the "scientific," systematic, approach to data collection, analysis, and interpretation that can be validated by more than researchers themselves; on the other hand, the subjectivity position allows researchers to insert their personal and subjective interpretation into the research process.

Some scholars of autoethnography have also been pulled into the war. A special issue of *Journal of Contemporary Ethnography*, dedicated to autoethnography, illustrates the divide. In an article on "analytic autoethnography," Anderson (2006) leans toward the objectivity camp. The autoethnography that he advocates is expected to satisfy the following conditions: the autoethnographer (1) is "a complete member in the social world under study" (p. 379); (2) engages reflexivity to analyze data on self; (3) is visibly and actively present in the text; (4) includes other informants in similar situations in data collection; and (5) is committed to theoretical analysis. Atkinson (2006) aligns himself with Anderson's analytical, theoretical, and objective approach to autoethnography, whereas Ellis and Bochner (2006) and Denzin (2006) stand on the opposing end, arguing for "evocative" and emotionally engaging, more subjective autoethnography. Although some scholars straddle both positions (Best, 2006), this war between objectivity and subjectivity is likely to continue, shaping the discourse of autoethnography.

What Is Autoethnography?

Because autoethnography could mean different things to different people, I must clarify what I mean by autoethnography. The autoethnography that I promote in this book combines cultural analysis and interpretation with narrative details. It follows the anthropological and social scientific inquiry approach rather than descriptive or performative storytelling. That is, I expect the stories of autoethnographers to be reflected upon, analyzed, and interpreted within their broader sociocultural context.

Ellis and Bochner (2000) define autoethnography as "autobiographies that self-consciously explore the interplay of the introspective, personally engaged self with cultural descriptions mediated through language, history, and ethnographic explanation" (p. 742). Although their definition appears to focus more on autobiographical description than ethnographic analysis and interpretation—which I will discuss later in the book—they certainly acknowledge the importance of "ethnographic explanation." This "explanation" aspect makes autoethnography transcend autobiography by "connecting the personal to the cultural" (p. 739). The importance of linking "the self and the social" in autoethnography is also affirmed in Reed-Danahay's (1997) influential book, *Auto/Ethnography: Rewriting the Self and the Social*.

In the contemporary use of autoethnography, "self" connotes the ethnographer self. However, when the term "auto-ethnography" was first introduced by an anthropologist Heider (1975), "self" meant not the ethnographer but, rather, informants. In his study of the Dani people, he refers to their cultural accounts of themselves as Dani autoethnography. Hayano (1979) later used "autoethnography" in a yet different way to refer to a study of the ethnographer's "own people." His own people, in this case, are card players who spent "leisure hours playing cards in Southern California's legitimate card rooms" (Wolcott, 2004, p. 98). Hayano (1982) identified himself with this card-playing culture; this is his autobiographical connection to the ethnography.

Since then, a variety of labels have been used to refer to autoethnographic applications in social science research. For Reed-Danahay, the label of autoethnography embraces a broad scope of writings such as (1) "native anthropology," in which members of previously studied cultural groups become ethnographers of their own groups; (2) "ethnic autobiography," in which personal narratives are written by members of ethnic minority groups; and (3) "autobiographical ethnography," in which anthropologists interject personal experience into ethnographic writing (p. 2).

Ellis and Bochner (2000), scholars of communication arts, present an even wider array of labels that indicate an autoethnographic orientation. The labels include (pp. 739–740). [1]

autobiographical ethnography
autobiology
auto-observation
autopathography
collaborative autobiography
complete-member research
confessional tales
critical autobiography
emotionalism narratives of the self
ethnobiography
ethnographic autobiography
ethnographic memoir
ethnographic poetics
ethnographic short stories
evocative narratives
experiential texts
first-person accounts
impressionistic accounts
indigenous ethnography
interpretive biography
literary tales
lived experience

narrative ethnography
native ethnography
new or experimental ethnography
opportunistic research
personal essays
personal ethnography
personal experience narrative
personal narratives
personal writing
postmodern ethnography
radical empiricism
reflexive ethnography
self-ethnography
self-stories
socioautobiography
sociopoetics
writing-stories

Having grown out of various disciplines, the variety reflects diverging evolution of this genre.

These autoethnographic terms and labels put different emphases on self and the ethnographic process. Even those claimed as "auto-ethnography" do not balance autobiography and ethnography in the same way. Ellis and Bochner (2000) offer an insightful triadic model to explain the complexity of the autoethnographic variety. They observe that "[a]utoethnographers vary in their emphasis on the research process (graphy), on culture (ethno), and on self (auto)" and that "[d]ifferent exemplars of autoethnography fall at different places along the continuum of each of these three axes" (p. 740). Keeping in mind the triadic balance, I argue that autoethnography should be ethnographic in its methodological orientation, cultural in its interpretive orientation, and autobiographical in its content orientation.

These three aspects make autoethnography similar to and different from other ethnographies. First, like ethnographers, autoethnographers follow a similar ethnographic research process by systematically collecting data, "field texts" in Clandinin and Connelly's (2000) words, analyzing and interpreting them, and producing scholarly reports, also called autoethnography. In this sense, the term "autoethnography" refers to the process and the product, just as "ethnography" does. Second, like ethnographers, autoethnographers attempt to achieve cultural understanding through analysis and interpretation. In other words, autoethnography is not about focusing on self alone, but about searching for understanding of others (culture/society) through self. Thus, self is a subject to look into and a lens to look through to gain an understanding of a societal culture (Duckart, 2005). The last aspect of autoethnography sets it apart from other ethnographic inquiries. Autoethnographers use their personal experiences as primary data. The richness of autobiographical narratives and autobiographical insights is valued and intentionally integrated in the research process and product unlike conventional ethnography. As Muncey (2005) states, "Autoethnography celebrates rather than demonizes the individual story" (p. 2). Yet, individual stories are framed in the context of the bigger story, a story of the society, to make autoethnography ethnographic.

What I focus on in this book is autoethnographies that are ethnographic in their intent and that utilize basic ethnographic and "narrative inquiry" approaches (Clandinin & Connelly, 2000). Like ethnography, autoethnography pursues the ultimate goal of cultural understanding underlying autobiographical experiences. To achieve this ethnographic intent, autoethnographers undergo the usual ethnographic research process of data collection, data analysis/interpretation, and report writing. They collect field data by means of participation, observation, interview, and document review; verify data by triangulating sources and contents from multiple origins; analyze and interpret data to decipher the cultural meanings of events, behaviors, and thoughts; and write ethnography. Like ethnographers, autoethnographers are expected to treat their autobiographical data with critical, analytical, and interpretive eyes to detect cultural undertones of what is recalled, observed, and told. At the end of a thorough self-examination in its cultural context, autoethnographers hope to gain a cultural understanding of self and others directly and indirectly connected to self.

Autoethnographic Research Focus

As in any other research endeavor, autoethnographers face the initial challenge of identifying a research focus: what to study. And as in ethnographic research, an initial focus will be refined, often narrowed, and sometimes redirected in the course of study. This does not mean that researchers can take the initial step of identifying a research focus carelessly. For autoethnography, virtually any aspect of one's life can become a research focus. Some researchers may focus on a broad scope of their lives (e.g., growing up Korean) while others may select more specific topics in their lives (e.g., the Korean female identity).

Some topics may be more emotive and personal and others not. One difference between ethnography and autoethnography at the initial stage is that autoethnographers enter the research field with a familiar topic (self) whereas ethnographers begin their investigation with an unfamiliar topic (others).

A variety of topics have been explored in book-length, chapter-length, and article-length autoethnographies. Ellis's *Final Negotiations* (1995), Nash's *Spirituality, Ethics, Religion, and Teaching* (2002), and Tompkins's *A Life in School* (1996) are examples of full-length books drawing from the broad scope of the authors' lives. Although only Ellis explicitly labeled her work an "autoethnography," Nash's and Tompkins's writings have an autoethnographic quality. All discuss the professorial culture either primarily or tangentially. Ellis's description of her professorial life is intertwined with her account of her partnership with another academician, the illness and eventual death of her partner, and her grief over the loss. Nash's "scholarly personal narrative" contains his personal reflection like Ellis's, but his focus is more straightforwardly on his intellectual journey beginning with graduate study and eventually reaching the height of seasoned professorship. Compared to Nash's, Tompkins's academic memoir covers a wider span of her life, beginning with childhood; she addresses her school experience first as a student and later as a professor. In addition to such book-length coverage encompassing a broad scope of the autoethnographer's life, many autoethnographies that focus more narrowly on a life have been published in book-chapter length (see chapters in Reed-Danahay, 1997; Ellis & Bochner, 1996; Bochner & Ellis, 2002) or journal-article length (see the next paragraph). In the 2000s, articles labeled autoethnography become noticeable in qualitative research journals such as *International Journal of Qualitative Methods, Journal of Contemporary Ethnography, Symbolic Interaction,* and *Qualitative Inquiry.*

Article-length autoethnographic studies frequently cover emotive topics, sometimes including those conventionally kept private, such as a complex mother-daughter relationship (Ellis, 1996), a father's death (Wyatt, 2005), childhood with a psychotic parent (Foster, McAllister, & O'Brien, 2005), childhood with a "mentally retarded" mother (Ronai, 1996), motherhood with a schizophrenic child (Schneider, 2005), child sexual abuse (Fox, 1996), teenage pregnancy (Muncey, 2005), domestic abuse (Olson, 2004), bulimia (Tillmann-Healy, 1996), brain injury (Smith, 2005), stroke (Kelley & Betsalel, 2004), chronic pain (Neville-Jan, 2003), and illness (Ettorre, 2005). These personal topics fit autoethnographic inquiries well because researchers have direct access to intimate information and can investigate the subjects in depth. Especially in the medical/nursing field where patient privacy concerns limit researcher access, autoethnography becomes a viable option. Although this uniquely personal, frequently private approach to autoethnography has been criticized as being narcissistic or self-indulgent (Holt, 2003; Salzman, 2002; Sparkes, 2002), Bochner and Ellis (2002) do not apologize for the personal nature of this inquiry, but rather boldly promote its therapeutic effect on authors and readers. I agree that such emotive autoethnographies powerfully engage readers in a meaningful understanding of the autoethnographer's personal and societal context. At the same time, I argue that mere self-exposure without profound cultural analysis and interpretation leaves this writing at the level of descriptive autobiography or memoir.

Not all autoethnographic topics are concerned with the sensitive realm of private life. Examples of less sensitive topics include mother-daughter relationship (Ellis, 1996), father-son relationship (Herrmann, 2005), female adolescence (Baker, 2001), Jewish identity (Edelman, 1996; Motzafi-Haller, 1997), Black identity (Austin, 1996), White-Chinese biraciality combined with African American cultural identity (Chin, 2006), Black-White multiculturality (Gatson, 2003), Cuban exile identity (Cotanda, 2006), White privilege (Magnet, 2006), military service as a female helicopter air navigator in the Canadian Forces (Taber, 2005), gender identity (Lucal, 1999), career change (Humphreys, 2005), and student teaching (Attard & Armour, 2005). In addition to these self-centric autoethnographies, Quinney (1996) and Brettell (1997) selected his father and her mother as subjects of their respective autoethnographies. Unlike these printed examples, Kim (2000) explores autoethnographic films produced by Korean adoptee filmmakers.

As I have illustrated here in Part I, all aspects of life can become a subject of autoethnography. When a research topic is selected, the most important question should be what to do with it. The minimum requirement is that autoethnographers must be willing to dig deeper into their memories, excavate rich details, bring them onto examination tables to sort, label, interconnect, and contextualize them in the sociocultural environment. Commitment to cultural analysis and interpretation is the key in proceeding with any topic.

Benefits of Autoethnography[2]

Autoethnography is becoming a particularly useful and powerful tool for researchers and practitioners who deal with human relations in multicultural settings, such as educators, social workers, medical professionals, clergy, and counselors. The benefits of autoethnography lie in three areas: (1) it offers a research method friendly to researchers and readers; (2) it enhances cultural understanding of self and others; and (3) it has a potential to transform self and others to motivate them to work toward cross-cultural coalition building.

Methodologically speaking, autoethnography is researcher-friendly. This inquiry method allows researchers easy access to the primary data source from the beginning because the source is the researchers themselves. In addition, autoethnographers are privileged with a holistic and intimate perspective on their "familiar data." This initial familiarity gives autoethnographers an edge over other researchers in data collection and in-depth data analysis/interpretation.

Autoethnography is also reader-friendly in that the personally engaging writing style tends to appeal to readers more than conventional scholarly writing. According to Nash (2004), "scholarly personal narratives" liberate researchers from abstract, impersonal writings and "touch readers' lives by informing their experiences" (p. 28). Gergen and Gergen (2002) also eloquently state, "In using oneself as an ethnographic exemplar, the researcher is freed from the traditional conventions of writing. One's unique voicing—complete with colloquialisms, reverberations from multiple relationships, and emotional expressiveness—is honored" (p. 14). This unique voice of the autoethnographer is a voice to which readers respond.

Second, autoethnography is an excellent vehicle through which researchers come to understand themselves and others. I have found this benefit particularly applicable to my teaching of multicultural education. As a teacher educator, I feel compelled to prepare my students to become cross-culturally sensitive and effective teachers for students of diverse cultural backgrounds. Self-reflection and self-examination are the keys to self-understanding (Florio-Ruane, 2001; Nieto, 2003). Kennett (1999) concurs with other advocates of self-reflection, saying that "[writing cultural] autobiography allows students to reflect on the forces that have shaped their character and informed their sense of self" (p. 231). The "forces" that shape people's sense of self include nationality, religion, gender, education, ethnicity, socioeconomic class, and geography. Understanding "the forces" also helps them examine their preconceptions and feelings about others, whether they are "others of similarity," "others of difference," or even "others of opposition" (Chang, 2005).

Not only writing one's own autoethnography but also reading others' autoethnographies can evoke self-reflection and self-examination (Florio-Ruane, 2001; Nash, 2002). Connelly shares a poignant story of how reading the self-narrative of his doctoral student of Chinese heritage stirred up his childhood memory of a Chinese store owner from his rural hometown in Canada (Clandinin & Connelly, 2000). Through self-reflection, he discovered shared humanity between this stranger of his childhood and himself. This discovery of self and others is a definite benefit of doing and sharing autoethnographies.

Third, doing, sharing, and reading autoethnography can also help transform researchers and readers (listeners) in the process. The transformation of self and others may not always be a conscious goal of autoethnography. Berry (2006) is not even sure if the evocative nature of the highly personal autoethnographic discourse is always a "gift" to the audience or readers who do not know how to respond to emotional provocation or are not willing to subject themselves to inadvertent conversion. However, personal engagement in auto-ethnographic stories frequently stirs the self-reflection of listeners, a powerful by-product of this research inquiry. Coia and Taylor's (2006) experimentation with "co/autoethnography" illustrates this benefit. In this participatory process, the researchers involved their education students in writing personal narratives, meeting in small groups weekly to share the narratives aloud and collaborate on a cultural analysis, exchanging newly acquired self-awareness on "their past, present, and future selves," and ultimately "strengthen[ing] perspective on teaching" (p. 21). In the end, the authors witnessed that students' self-awareness and cultural understanding were broadened and their teaching philosophies and practices became more inclusive and sensitive to others' needs.

Self-transformation may be manifested in a variety of ways in the education field. Some may become more self-reflective in their daily praxis (Florio-Ruane, 2001; Nieto, 2004; Obidah & Teel, 2001). Others may adopt "culturally relevant pedagogy" when selecting curriculum content and pedagogical strategies and interacting with students, peer teachers, and the community (Ladson-Billings, 1994). Self-transformation may also take place as educators seek to reach out to unfamiliar others and pursue a new learning of unfamiliar cultures. As their understanding of others increases, unfamiliarity diminishes and perspectives on others change. As a result, others of difference and of opposition may be reframed to be included in their notion of community, "extended community" in Greene's (2000) term.

Another type of self-transformation may bring about healings from the emotional scars of the past, which Foster illuminated in her writing (Foster, McAllister, & O'Brien, 2005). By sharing with others her painful experience of growing up with a mother with schizophrenia and understanding the cultural root of her "wounds,"

Foster experienced liberation and relief from the burden of isolation, loneliness, and shame. The liberating force of autoethnography was the foundation of self-empowerment for Foster.

When manifested in increased self-reflection, adoption of the culturally relevant pedagogy, desire to learn about "others of difference," development of an inclusive community, or self-healing, the self-transformative potential of autoethnography is universally beneficial to those who work with people from diverse cultural backgrounds. Through the increased awareness of self and others, they will be able to help themselves and each other correct cultural misunderstandings, develop cross-cultural sensitivity, and respond to the needs of cultural others effectively.

Pitfalls to Avoid in Doing Autoethnography

In the shadow of the growing interest in and support of auto-ethnographic research methods, criticism is lurking. The scrutiny of autoethnography is illustrated by peer reviews that Holt (2003) received on her submission of an autoethnographic manuscript. Reviewers questioned the academic rigor and methodological validity and claimed to detect subjectivity. Such criticism does not necessarily imply that autoethnography is inherently faulty. Even so, it is always helpful to look out vigilantly for appropriate application of this research inquiry and avoid potential pitfalls. Here are five potential pitfalls that autoethnographers need to watch out for: (1) excessive focus on self in isolation from others; (2) overemphasis on narration rather than analysis and cultural interpretation; (3) exclusive reliance on personal memory and recalling as a data source; (4) negligence of ethical standards regarding others in self-narratives; and (5) inappropriate application of the label "autoethnography."

The first pitfall relates to the very notion of culture. In the minds of anthropologists, culture is inherently a group-oriented concept. Culture and people have a symbiotic relationship, on which I elaborated in Chapter 1. Therefore, the notion of *culture* predisposes the co-presence of others even in a discussion of "individual culture." Autoethnography, therefore, should reflect the interconnectivity of self and others. Unfortunately, the methodological focus on self is sometimes misconstrued as a license to dig deeper in personal experiences without digging wider into the cultural context of the individual stories commingled with others. Autoethnographers should be warned that self-indulgent introspection is likely to produce a self-exposing story but not autoethnography.

Second, autoethnographers swept by the power of storytelling can easily neglect the very important mission of autoethnography—cultural interpretation and analysis of autobiographic texts (Reed-Danahay, 1997). Wall (2006) articulates the autoethnographic intent as "to acknowledge the inextricable link between the personal and the cultural and to make room for nontraditional forms of inquiry and expression." Self-narration is very engaging to writers as well as readers and listeners (Foster, McAllister, & O'Brien, 2005; Nash, 2004; Tompkins, 1996). Yet, as Coia and Taylor (2006) say, "It is not enough simply to tell the story or write a journal entry" (p. 19) for the cultural understanding of self to take place. Unless autoethnographers stay focused on their research purpose, they can be tempted to settle for elaborate narratives with underdeveloped cultural analysis and interpretation.

Third, autoethnographers can fall into the pitfall of over-relying on their personal memory as the source of data. Personal memory is a marvelous and unique source of information for autoethnographers. It taps into the reservoir of data to which other ethnographers have no access. Yet, Muncey (2005) reminds us, "Memory is selective and shaped, and is retold in the continuum of one's experience, [although] this does not necessarily constitute lying" (p. 2). Memory can censor past experiences. When data are collected from a single tool without other measures for checks and balances, the validity of data can be questioned. When the single tool is the researcher self, the unbridled subjectivity of autoethnographers can be more severely challenged (Holt, 2003). Although an obsession with objectivity is not necessary for qualitative research, autoethnographers need to support their arguments with broad-based data as in any good research practice. For this reason, they can easily complement "internal" data generated from researchers' memory with "external" data from outside sources, such as interviews, documents, and artifacts. Multiple sources of data can provide bases for triangulation that will help enhance the content accuracy and validity of the autoethnographic writing.

The fourth pitfall stems from a false notion that confidentiality does not apply to self-narrative studies because researchers use their autobiographical stories. Playing the multi-faceted role of researcher, informant, and author, autoethnographers may be tempted to claim full authorship and responsibility for their stories without hesitation. Clandinin and Connelly's (2000) poignant question to narrative inquirers, "Do they own a story because they tell it?" should equally challenge autoethnographers. Since autoethnographers' personal stories are often linked to stories of others, no matter how explicit the linkage is, the principle of protecting confidentiality of people in the story is just as relevant to autoethnography. Because main characters reveal their identities in autoethnography, it is extremely difficult to fully protect others intimately connected to these known characters. Yet, autoethnographers, like other researchers of human subjects, are charged with adhering to the ethical principle of confidentiality. This inquiry method requires researchers to adopt creative strategies in practicing the principle.

The last pitfall concerns the confusion in use of the term "auto-ethnography." As I discussed earlier in the chapter, the term has been used to refer to a variety of narrative inquiries that have sprung up in different academic disciplines. The mixed bag labeled autoethnography has confused researchers as well as readers. Since no one can claim an exclusive license to use this label, researchers have the responsibility to become informed of the multiple usage of the term and to define their choice clearly to avoid confusion. That is precisely what Wolcott (2004) does in his article "Ethnographic Autobiography." Although my use of autoethnography differs from what he proposes—leaving the term to the original meaning by Hayano who refers to autoethnography as a study of the researcher's own people—his conscious clarification of the term clearly orients readers. With the rigorous effort to distinguish autoethnography from other self-narrative inquiries, readers will be able to understand this research method by what it stands for, distinguishing it from highly descriptive self-narratives such as auto-biography and memoir.

Summary

This chapter presents autoethnography as a qualitative research method that utilizes ethnographic methods to bring cultural interpretation to the autobiographical data of researchers with the intent of under-standing self and its connection to others. This research method stems from the long-standing anthropological interest in self but has spread to other social science fields. The long list of autoethnographic labels and terms, presented in Ellis and Bochner (2000), indicates that the social scientists' interest in self has increased significantly. This book will limit its consideration to autoethnographies that handle auto-biographical data with ethnographic methodology and intent. Research topics that autoethnographers have investigated are diverse, from more personal to less personal topics, from emotive to emotionally distanced topics, and from a broad scope of life to more narrowly focused aspects of life. When a personally meaningful topic is chosen and investigation is contextualized appropriately in the sociocultural context of the researcher, autoethnography can powerfully engage readers in understanding not only the autoethnographers' worlds but also others in them.

Reading and writing autoethnography present a variety of benefits. The self-reflection can lead to self-transformation through self-understanding. The cultural understanding of self and others has the potential of cross-cultural coalition building. Methodologically speaking, the direct access to autobiographical data provides researchers with the possibility of reaching the height of holistic and in-depth cultural self-analysis quickly.

Although autoethnography has many benefits, it can also become a research method with little social impact if several pitfalls are not carefully avoided. They include (1) excessive focus on self in isolation from others; (2) overemphasis on narration rather than analysis and cultural interpretation; (3) exclusive reliance on personal memory and recalling as a data source; (4) negligence of ethical standards regarding others in self-narratives; and (5) inappropriate application of the label "autoethnography." Given a clear understanding that autoethnography is a rigorous ethnographic, broadly qualitative research method that attempts to achieve in-depth cultural understanding of self and others, this inquiry has much to offer to social scientists, especially those concerned with raising cross-cultural understanding in a culturally diverse society.

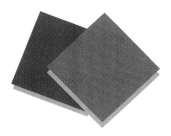

Part II
Collecting Autoethnographic Data

Having read the theoretical discussions of culture, self-narratives, and autoethnography in Part I, you may be eager to begin an autoethnographic study of your life. In Part II, I present practical methodological guidance to help you collect a variety of data from yourself and others. As you read Chapter 4, think through four rudimentary questions to get started with your study: why you want to undertake an autoethnographic study, how you can find a research focus, what initial steps you need to take in your study, and how you should handle ethical concerns. During the initial steps of research, many more questions, such as how you can gather your autobiographical data, will come to you.

Chapters 5 through 7 address these questions by detailing types of data that you can collect and methodological strategies for collecting those data. Chapter 5 suggests chronicling, inventorying, and visualizing self as strategies for capturing personal memory data. These data involve not only you but also others from your family, local community, and broader society, who have been enmeshed in your life. In Chapter 6 you will focus on data from your present. Utilizing systematic self-observation, the field journal, the culture-gram, and self-analysis, you will be able to collect self-observational and self-reflective data. Whereas Chapters 5 and 6 direct you toward data from within yourself, Chapter 7 guides your attention to data collection from external sources: for example, textual and nontextual artifacts, interviews with others, and literature pertaining to your research topic or your cultures. These external sources provide contextual information to your autoethnography and additional data with which you can validate and triangulate memory-based and self-reflective data.

Getting Ready

Autoethnographic research takes careful planning like any other research design. Given that autoethnography is more than casually recalled and accounted memories, your research plan needs to delineate why and how you want to explore your own life and what you want to explore in it. The *why*-question helps you articulate a research *purpose*: Why do you want to undertake a study of yourself, and what is the goal you intend to accomplish at the end of the research process? The *what*-question guides you to narrow a research *topic*: What do you intend to study in your life? When the goal and direction of a study are clear in your mind, you are ready to ask *how*-questions: How will you collect data about yourself and integrate others in your study? How will you manage, analyze, and interpret data? How will you present research outcomes? These process-oriented questions form the backbone of subsequent methodology chapters.

While wrestling with why, what, and how questions, you should keep in mind that the ethnographic research process is never neatly linear or sequential. Research steps often overlap and mix. For example, even after a research focus is set, it is possible for the focus to be modified and refined while data are being collected; collected data are used to validate the research focus or alter your research direction. Data analysis begins while data collection is still in progress, and analysis facilitates the collection of more relevant and meaningful data. Ethnographic writing often concurs with data analysis and interpretation, and this dynamic process sometimes spurs more data collection. This multi-layered ethnographic process allows the research focus to be sharpened, relevant data to be collected, and in-depth interpretation to be applied along the way. Following this principle of ethnography, autoethnographic research design also defies a rigid and linear model of research design.

How to Find Research Topics

Autoethnography uses self as the subject of investigation. If you are interested in studying yourself and are convinced of the benefits of this research method laid out in Chapter 3, autoethnography could be for you. Culture is complex and multi-dimensional. An autoethnography, therefore, can cover a broad spectrum of your culture, as anthropologist Mead (1972) did in her autobiography.[1] Yet exploring your culture holistically can be a daunting task because the subject is vast and complex. Zooming in on a narrow dimension of life may give an attractive alternative for rookie autoethnographers and for the experienced who intend to conduct a small-scale, perhaps article-length, autoethnography.

You may approach the task of identifying a narrow topic to study in one of two ways: the specific-to-general and the general-to-specific. The specific-to-general approach starts with some specifics from your life such as memorable experiences, repeated events, or life routines. By looking into these specifics, you may discover thoughts or beliefs that persist, issues and concerns that envelop them, memories that surface to consciousness, or emotions that grip you firmly. By looking beyond the specifics of your life, you may identify others in a sustaining relationship with you, influential others in a positive and negative sense, or significant organizations/communities/nation that have supported your life. By looking into and beyond your specific experiences, you can generate a general research topic to explore.

Another way of finding a research topic uses the general-to-specific approach, which takes the matter in the opposite direction, beginning with a broad and general topic of interest and excavating personal experiences relating to the topic. General topics of interest may emerge as you review literature, consult with experienced researchers, or pick the brains of your colleagues.

A literature review is highly rated as the main source of research ideas, especially at the initial stage of research. Although the literature review is not emphasized as much in qualitative research as in quantitative research as a means to find research topics or to legitimize your study, the presence of a literature review in qualitative research textbooks still attests to the love affair between researchers and this convention (Bogdan & Biklen, 2003; Creswell, 2003; Maxwell, 2005; Silverman, 2000). There is a reason for the love affair. Searching through literature, you can indeed discover well-researched concepts, ideas that match your interest, or less-well-explored topics that are worthy of further investigation.

The literature review helps you validate a research topic that has emerged from your personal experiences. Foster (Foster, McAllister, & O'Brien, 2005) used literature this way. After she was inspired to investigate her personal experience of growing up with a mother suffering from paranoid schizophrenia, she undertook a literature review, through which she discovered that much research had been done on this general topic by outsiders (those who do not have personal experiences), but not enough by insiders. So she decided to pursue a study involving her own experience as an "insider" researcher. She describes the literature review as a process of professional validation of a research idea drawn from her personal experience:

> During this process of discovery, in finding there was literature and research on an aspect of my life that I had previously borne in silence and largely alone, I felt a sense of wonder. I find it hard to describe the amazement that came with discovering that others actually knew about, and had acknowledged and validated through research, the impact of being the child of a parent with mental illness. (Foster, McAllister, & O'Brien, p. 4)

Although many researchers resort to literature in search of good research topics, the value of talking to others—experienced researchers and peers—cannot be underestimated. The dialogical exchange of ideas often helps generate ideas for further investigation. Foster's research idea initially resulted from her personal conversation with a friend and subsequently with her dissertation advisor who helped her connect dots between her life experience and research. Her advisor posed the following questions that evoked more introspection within Foster:

— How does your life experience shape the theory that will frame your method?
— What "cultural baggage" do you bring to the research encounter?

— How might this research endeavor be emancipatory/transformative for you? . . .
— What issues are likely to be strange/familiar for you when you encounter [others in a similar situation]?
— How will your identity place limitations on the research?
— How will your identity offer opportunities, insights, [and] innovations for the research? And for the readers of your research?

— In what ways does this raised awareness of your identity help to bring into focus the relationship between the researcher and [others in the similar situation]? . . .
— How do people react to you when you declare/have declared this identity? (Foster, McAllister, & O'Brien, p. 2)

Some of these questions are more relevant to Foster et al.'s study than to others', yet many of the questions can be useful to general autoethnographic research.

At this stage, I suggest that you list five broad topics of interest to you, from which a final topic may be selected for your autoethnography, and then rate each topic by four criteria: personal interest, professional significance, manageability, and ethical consideration. *Personal interest* refers to how passionately you feel about the topic, how enduring it is to you, and how invested you are. *Professional significance* indicates how this topic may contribute to your professional development and the advancement of your professional discipline. *Manageability* is an important consideration because it is largely responsible for the success of any research. No project is inherently more manageable or difficult than another. It depends on your research readiness, resources, data accessibility, timeline, and other systematic constraints. Although changed circumstances can alter the level of manageability, you may want to assess your current situation appropriately to determine the manageability of your topic. The last, but not least, consideration is *ethical standards*. As I discussed in Chapter 3, ethical consideration applies to autoethnography in which you involve others as the source of data or as co-participants in your study (Berger & Ellis, 2007). Evaluate each topic by these criteria and assign five points for the highest possibility and one point for the lowest possibility. Calculate an aggregate score for each topic. If a certain criterion is more important to you, I suggest you double the score of that criterion before calculating the total score. In my teaching of research design, this method has helped my students think systematically in this initial process of research. Not all students stick with the highest-scoring topic for their final project. Yet this process, albeit simple and quantitative, seems to make this overwhelming first step more manageable, especially for novice researchers.

Where to Position Self and Others in Autoethnography

Given that culture is a web of self and others, autoethnography is not a study simply of self alone. Others personally or conceptually connected to self are often incorporated in autoethnography. Family members, friends, colleagues, and neighbors are others personally connected to self. Strangers can be connected to self through group membership or common experiences, if not through personal contacts. In autoethnography, self and others may be positioned in different ways. You can consider three possibilities. First, you can investigate yourself as a main character and others as supporting actors in your life story. Second, you can include others as co-participants or co-informants in your study. Third, you can study others as the primary focus, yet also as an entry to your world.

The first approach seems most common in autoethnography: The life of self is the primary focus of inquiry, and others are explored only in auxiliary relationships with self. Studies by Lazarre (1996), Nash (2002), Tillmann-Healy (1996), and Tompkins (1996) fall into this category. Lazarre explores her parenting experience as a White mother raising White-Black biracial sons; Nash discusses how his professorial role has evolved; Tillmann-Healy focuses on her affliction with bulimia; and Tompkins exposes her educational experiences. In all of them, authors are the main narrators, interpreters, and researchers of their personal experiences. Lazarre's sons, Nash's mentor and students, Tillmann-Healy's mother, and Tompkins's colleagues and family members play the roles of supporting actors occupying the fringe of these authors' stories as others of similarity or difference.

In the second approach, you may decide to investigate a certain life experience of yours, but, instead of studying only yourself, you include others with a similar experience as co-participants in your study. This approach broadens the database by including others of similarity, but the research focus is still anchored in your personal experience. Foster, McAllister, and O'Brien (2005) and Smith (2005) adopted this approach. Foster et al.'s study was inspired by the first author's personal experience of growing up with a mother suffering from paranoid schizophrenia. Foster's personal experience is thoroughly reflected upon, and others' experiences are utilized as an equally important source of data. So, self and others are equally emphasized and valued as Foster and her co-authors use "self as the starting point for the study and for inclusion in field text analysis alongside the experiences of the participants." (Foster, McAllister, & O'Brien, 2005, p.5). Smith (2005) also adopted this approach when she included herself as the fifth participant in her study exploring "the impact of creativity on the self-esteem of individuals who have sustained ABIs [acquired brain injuries]." Her personal experience as an ABI survivor added a unique perspective to her autoethnography of healing.

The third approach is not noted as autoethnography by Ellis and Bochner (2000) for a probably legitimate reason. It does not engage self sufficiently to earn the label of autoethnography. Yet it is common in social science research, in that researchers use their personal experiences or perspectives to guide the selection of their research topic or subjects without centering on self. In this approach, self opens a door to an investigation but remains outside while others are in the spotlight as main characters or participants. Bateson (1994), Brettell (1997), and Kikumura (1981) explored lives of their parents: respectively, renowned anthropologist parents Margaret Mead and Gregory Bateson, a journalist mother, and an immigrant mother from Japan. In both Crane's (2000) study of Jewish wives of Christians who survived the Holocaust in Nazi Germany and Frankenberg's (1993) study of White women in interracial liaison with Black men, authors do not expose their personal experiences explicitly but use their personal connection to the topic as a springboard to their study. Although these authors do not investigate their lives per se, the cultural analyses of their family members or others of similarity invariably shed a light on the authors' own lives.

Once you understand these variable positions of self in auto-ethnographic studies, you may want to consider the question of why you want to study yourself. Is it because you want to make cultural sense of yourself, to use your story as part of a larger study of others, or to investigate a topic dear to your personal experience without centering on yourself? Where you position yourself in your study will affect your research design.

How to Proceed from Here

When your research purpose and focus are identified, you are ready to ask further questions: How should I go about getting information on the determined research topic, how should I analyze and interpret the gathered information, and how should I present the outcome?

These *how* questions frame the steps of methodological planning. The first question is about data collection—what, where, how, and with whom to collect data. Ethnographic data are primarily text-based, rather than number-based. The majority of textual data are likely to be generated by researchers in the form of field notes, journals, and interview transcripts. Other textual data come from external sources through official documents, personal writings by others, and published literature. In addition to textual data, a variety of non-textual data—multimedia, artifacts, audio-recording, and graphic images—can be collected. The next three chapters are dedicated to practical data collection techniques. Although a data collection plan in a qualitative study, including autoethnography, can be easily modified throughout the research process, having a basic plan of data collection from the outset enhances the effectiveness and efficiency of an autoethnographic study.

Planning the subsequent step—data analysis and interpretation—is more difficult because data analysis and interpretation hinge on data collection, often not prescribed by a rigid research design. Once you understand the fluidity of the process, you can design a flexible plan to analyze and interpret data, some techniques of which are explained in Chapter 9.

Writing an autoethnography seems a remote concern at this point of research design. Without content to write about and with the fear of influencing the research process with preconceived notions of predicted outcomes, you may be inclined to ignore the careful planning of a writing strategy. However, one of the best pieces of advice I received from my doctoral advisor many years ago is that I should think early on about what the finished writing would look like. Of course, the table of contents I drafted at the planning stage of my ethnographic study did not look at all like what it was at the end (Chang, 1992a). Nevertheless, however crude and drafty it was, the initial table of contents gave me a basic framework to work with, to reconsider, and to sharpen. The evolution of my table of contents illustrates the flexibility of qualitative research design. Not a rigid design, but a keen observation of a malleable process produces an insightful interpretation of a phenomenon you set out to explore.

The flexibility of research design should not be misconstrued as a lack of diligence or indecisiveness in planning. Rather, this research design gives you freedom to modify your plan as needed so that the most insightful understanding of complex human experiences can be gained with few presumptions and an open mind. Thus, auto-ethnographic research planning needs to reflect this principle.

Ethical Issues

Since most autoethnographies focus primarily on self, you may feel that ethical issues involving human subjects do not apply to your research design. This assumption is incorrect. Whichever format you may take, you still need to keep in mind that other people are always present in self-narratives, either as active participants in the story or as associates in the background (Morse, 2002). If your study engages others as interviewees or the observed, you should treat your study in the same way as other social science research requiring an Institutional Review Board (IRB) approval. Even when you are the primary source of data, your story often includes others—others of similarity, difference, and/or opposition. Some of them are more intimately interwoven into your story than others who are mentioned only in passing. Therefore, it is advisable to check with the IRB of your learning institution about its approval requirements for autoethnographic research.

The IRB is "a committee made up of faculty members who review and approve research so that the rights of the participants are protected" (Creswell, 2002, p. 160). The creation of IRBs, required by "the OPRR published regulations (45 CFR 46), most recently revised in 1991" (Best & Kahn, 2003, p. 50), intends to oversee research processes to ensure that research practices adhere to the principles of "informed consent," "right to privacy," and "protection from harm" (Fontana & Frey, 2000, p. 662). "Informed consent" refers to "receiving consent by the subject after having carefully and truthfully informed him or her about the research"; "right to privacy," to "protecting the identity of the subject"; and "protection from harm," to protecting human subjects from "physical, emotional, or any other kind [of harms]."

Even when your research proposal is exempt from a formal review process, you should consider the code of confidentiality in all steps of your inquiry. Protecting the privacy of others in autoethnographic stories is much more difficult than in other studies involving human subjects. Because your identity is already disclosed, the identities of others connected to you sometimes become transparent to the broader audience and other times to smaller circles of your acquaintances. For example, Foster, McAllister, and O'Brien (2005) expose Foster's mother's psychosis by the natural mother-daughter association; Ronai's "retarded" mother (1996) and Olson's abusive ex-husband (2004) are also exposed to the public through the authors' writings. To protect the privacy of others connected to you, you might use pseudonyms for some or all, create composite figures based on factual details to obscure their identities, or let voices of others tell your story.

Morse (2002), Editor of *Qualitative Health Research*, suggested the use of a "publishing *nom de plume*" (p. 1159). If none of these options is ideal for you, you simply have to use the real identities of others with their consent. Although perfect protection of privacy is not always possible, you should model an honest and conscious effort to adhere to the ethical code of research.

Clandinin and Connelly (2000) challenge all self-narrative writers with a poignant question: "Do they own a story because they tell it?" As you play a multi-faceted role as researcher, informant, and author, you should be reminded that your story is never made in a vacuum and others are always visible or invisible participants in your story.

Summary

This chapter has laid out four initial steps that you need to consider as you undertake an autoethnographic study. First, identify a research topic, whether narrowly defined or multi-dimensional. Second, determine your position (role) in relation to others in your study. Will you be the primary subject of the study with others in the background? Will you include others along with yourself as co-participants in your study? Or will you study only others on the topic that has a personal connection to you? When the focus and topic are determined, you need to begin methodological planning for data collection, analysis, interpretation, and reporting. Along with the methodological design, you are expected to adhere to ethical standards of research to protect the privacy of human subjects involved in your study.

Having taken care of the preliminary planning, you are ready to delve into the practice of data collection, management, analysis, and interpretation. The following chapters in Part II are designed to help you experiment with different data collection strategies. With the understanding that ethnographic process is not rigidly sequential, you may mix and match strategies of data collection, analysis, and interpretation to find the ones that best serve your research goal.

Collecting Personal Memory Data

Personal memory is a building block of autoethnography because the past gives a context to the present self and memory opens a door to the richness of the past. As an autoethnographer, you not only have a privileged access to your past experiences and personal interpretations of those experiences, but also have first-hand discernment of what is relevant to your study. What is recalled from the past forms the basis of autoethnographic data.

"Recalling" in autoethnography is no different in principle from its practice in other ethnographies. Both you as an autoethnographer and ethnographers often rely on memory when collecting data. However, you and the ethnographers utilize different memories as the primary source of data and differently acknowledge the prominence of personal memory in research. Autoethnography values your personal memory, whereas ethnography relies on informants' personal memory and ethnographers' recent memory of what they observed and heard in the field. Another major difference between you and other ethnographers is that you openly acknowledge your personal memory as a primary source of information in your research. In contrast, most ethnographers avoid mixing their personal memories with their data collected from fieldwork.

Memory is not always a friend to autoethnography; it is sometimes a foe. It often reveals partial truth and is sometimes unreliable and unpredictable. Memory selects, shapes, limits, and distorts the past. Some distant memories remain vivid while other recent memories fade away quickly, blurring the time gap between these memories. In general, though, time tends to "smooth out details, leaving a kind of schematic landscape outline" (Dillard, cited in Clandinin & Connelly, 2000, p. 83). Reconstructing the details later is a challenging task, and the reliability of the outcome may be questioned. Memory can also trigger extreme emotions: aversion with an unpleasant experience and glorification of a pleasant one. For example, Ronai (1996) writes about her deep sense of resentment and embarrassment about her "mentally retarded" mother in her childhood. In comparison, Catherine Bateson (1994) romanticizes infrequent, but precious, meals that her anthropologist mother Margaret Mead prepared in her childhood. This seemingly aggrandized memory is in stark contrast with her otherwise lonesome childhood wrought by her mother's frequent fieldwork and professional engagement away from home.

Despite its precariousness, personal memory taps into the wealth of information on self. What is extracted through memory can be written down as textual data. In this chapter I will facilitate the collection of textual data from your past. Through writing exercises of chronicling, inventorying, and visualizing self, you are encouraged to unravel your memory, write down fragments of your past, and build the database for your cultural analysis and interpretation. As I reminded you earlier, writing exercises suggested here should be treated as catalysts for further thoughts. You are encouraged to expand on them to serve your own research purpose.

Chronicling the Past

The task of writing a self-narrative can be overwhelming when people try to tackle a complex and multi-faceted life as an entirety from the beginning. To help you better manage the autoethnographic research process, I suggest that you break it down to manageable steps. In the data collection stage, chronicling is a useful strategy through which you give a sequential order to bits of information you collect from memory. You can create an autobiographical timeline with memorable events or experiences in the order in which they happened in your lifetime or record the sequence of your personal and community routines. This strategy illuminates the evolution of your personal life and sequential regularity in your life.

Autobiographical Timeline

Your autobiographical timeline lists events or experiences from your life in chronological order. It can cover the whole span of life or a limited time period or stage of life. It can include all major events or only those relevant to a specific theme during a predetermined time span. The whole-life, all-major-event approach engenders the most comprehensive autobiographical timeline. Like other historical timelines, however, even the most comprehensive autobiographical timeline cannot contain every detail of life. You need to screen and select what to include. Your research focus is a good guidepost in the screening process.

A timeline useful for an autobiography, a life history, or a multi-faceted autoethnography is likely to focus on the whole life span. Centering on the theme of immigration, Kikumura (1981) wrote a life history of her immigrant mother. Beginning with her mother's childhood in Japan, the author describes subsequent phases of her mother's life as a picture bride who immigrated to marry a total stranger, a Japanese laborer living in the United States; as a pillar of a hard-working Asian immigrant family; as a Japanese resident in California who was declared a threat to national security and sent to an internment camp by the U.S. government during World War II; and as a postwar survivor building a once-lost life in the United States. Kikumura's own autobiographical timeline is interwoven into her mother's life history.

If you intend to create a thematically more focused timeline—your educational development, for example—you are likely to select your school experiences, educational accomplishments, and educational encounters for your autobiographical timeline. My Writing Sample 5.1.1 in Appendix B gives an example of my autobiographical timeline with an education focus. Such a timeline is likely to give a foundation to education-focused self-narratives like Tompkins's (1996) and Nash's (2002).

Another possible autobiographical timeline is one that zooms in on border-crossing experiences that occur when you become friends with others of difference or of opposition or when you place yourself in unfamiliar places or situations (e.g., visiting the home of someone from a different cultural background, learning a new language, and traveling in a foreign country). Such experiences with the unfamiliar cultural characteristics of others often challenge and cause you to adjust your cultural "standards" of thinking, perceiving, evaluating, and behaving (Goodenough, 1981, p. 62). Culturally speaking, these are significant moments of enlightenment, which often happen when you visit other countries (Lingenfelder, 1996).

A voluntary or involuntary removal from your cultural familiarities creates a "fish-out-of-water" sensation, which in turn contributes to self-discovery about what is familiar and strange to you (Hall, 1973). However, the sensation of cultural disconnection is not limited to national border-crossing. Your immediate environment sometimes engenders moments of disorientation when you step in an unfamiliar place, encounter others of difference, confront inequality between self and others, or are discriminated against for who you are. According to Helms and Cross, racial self-discovery is triggered by the dissonance that Blacks and Whites experience when they encounter inequality between themselves and the other race (Stephan, 1999). Transition from the pre-encounter stage to the encounter moment, when they become cognizant of their raciality, accelerates the journey of racial self-consciousness. Extraordinary events such as childbirth, new relationships, new jobs/schools, immigration/moves, a death, divorce, and other life crises also disrupt daily routines and challenge familiar values, which can lead to a new level of understanding of self and others. By chronicling border-crossing experiences, you will be able to see how your multicultural awareness has evolved in your lifetime. The Writing Sample 5.1.2 from Appendix B illustrates my example of an autobiographic timeline of border-crossing.

Consider the following writing exercise intended to help you create an autobiographical timeline as part of your personal memory data.

WRITING EXERCISE 5.1

Considering your research focus, select and chronologically list major events or experiences from your life. Include the date and brief account of each item. Select one event/experience from your timeline that led to significant cultural self-discovery. Describe its circumstances and explain why it is important in your life.

Annual, Seasonal, Weekly, or Daily Routines

While the autobiographical timeline documents extraordinary events or moments of life, routines represent the ordinariness of life. The life of an individual or a society is filled with routine activities or events repeated in a certain sequence and time cycle. Through annual, seasonal, weekly, or daily routines, people acquire language, customs, and traditions and become enculturated into patterns of a society. As society undergoes changes, some routines remain constant, others disappear, and new features emerge as new routines. Although personal and familial routines are not always synchronized with the rhythms of the broader society, their patterned routines of life are likely to reflect those of the culture in which individuals participate. Therefore, information on personal, familial, and societal routines is useful in discovering sociocultural patterns intertwined with your life, community, and society.

Some ethnographers use chronicling of life routines as a data collection strategy in their ethnographic studies. They observe and participate in chores, events, and celebrations repeated daily, weekly, seasonally, and annually in their informants' lives. For example, Wolcott's (2003b) chapter on a working day of an elementary school principal in his classic ethnography demonstrates the usefulness of this data collection strategy. In my ethnographic study of U.S. high school students (Chang, 1992a), I also elaborate on the daily routines of my female key informant from a semirural community.

Consider the following writing exercise, Writing Exercise 5.2 in Appendix B, to record routines of your life. Focus on one cycle of life and expand it to other cycles to broaden your database.

WRITING EXERCISE 5.2

Select a time cycle—annual, seasonal, weekly, or daily—that you want to focus on. List chronologically activities and/or events in which you participate regularly within this time cycle. Identify each item with the time framework (i.e., going to school at 7:00 am, going to church on Sunday, family visit in July/August, etc.). Briefly describe the context of such routines. Select one and describe it in detail.

In partial response to this writing exercise, I provide three writing samples in Appendix B: Writing Sample 5.2.1 on the annual routines in my professorial life, Writing Sample 5.2.2 on my weekly routines, and Writing Sample 5.2.3 on my typical teaching day.

Inventorying Self

During your autoethnographic research, you will collect lots of information bits. Some of them may appear more useful to your study than others at the time of collection. Even when you are guided by your research focus, however, you cannot help but feeling that they are just a bunch of disconnected bits. To avoid a total sense of randomness in your data collection, you may utilize inventorying as a starting activity. You may first consider your research focus and make a list of thematic categories relevant to your study. Then you rummage through the storehouse of your memory, pick up relevant bits of information on themes, and give an order to the thematically collected bits. In the process, you can expand your topics for inventory and add other information beyond your categories.

The inventory activity involves not only *collecting* but also *evaluating* and *organizing* data. You "collect" memory bits when recalling and writing them down. You evaluate and organize them by selecting and deselecting certain items and ranking them in the hierarchy of importance. Additional thematic categories for data collection may be born of this process of data evaluation and organization. Preliminary analysis and interpretation may also take place as you explain your selected items from your inventory lists. These multilayered activities open a door to future data analysis. The inventorying activity brings together data collection, analysis, and interpretation.

Here I suggest five thematic categories as a starter: proverbs, virtues and values, rituals, mentors, and artifacts. The categories can expand to represent the cognitive, affective, social, and material aspects of the culture that you have acquired in the interaction with others. For each writing exercise, I recommend that you select at least five items and prioritize them by their importance. The inventory writing exercises are similar to what Phifer (2002) refers to as "idea-gathering strategies." She suggests that lists be made regarding "people who have been important to you," "places where significant events in your life occurred," "things you have valued and would be sorry to lose," and "activities or experiences important to you" (pp. 21–23). After completing an inventory list of each category, you are encouraged to select one item and expound on it with details. The inventory lists and written texts drawn from your past become part of your personal memory data.

My five thematic categories and five items in each category are not set in stone. They should be taken as suggestions to initiate the process. You should feel limited neither by the number nor the particular thematic categories; rather, you should modify and expand these inventorying activities to meet your research needs.

Proverbs

A proverb is defined as "a condensed but memorable saying embodying some important fact of experience that is taken as true by many people" according to Wordnet Search 3.0 (Princeton University, 2006). Proverbs are said repeatedly and upheld by many to communicate their group wisdom and values. Through these, a group as small as a family transmits its values and regulates desirable and undesirable behaviors of its members.

Achebe's (1994) classic novel, *Things Fall Apart*, is full of proverbs through which readers are let into the world of Nigerian Ibo wisdom within which the author grew up. For example, "When the moon is shining the cripple becomes hungry for a walk" implies that it is acceptable that children play in open place on moonlit nights but not on dark nights (p. 11); "The Earth cannot punish me for obeying her messenger" connotes that it is safe to obey the Oracle (the spiritual leader of the clan) in all circumstances (p. 67).

Anderson (2000) also notes the importance of proverbs in Moroccan society. To explain Moroccans' social relationships, she introduces two proverbs: "A sin concealed is half-forgotten" and "Distrust your enemies once, but your friends a hundred times" (p. 104). The first proverb, she argues, communicates that Moroccans are expected to be highly attentive to relationships to others, more than to absolute moral standards from God or laws. The second proverb means, "Nor is there any inherent solace in a supportive group presence." Whether Anderson's interpretation of these proverbs fully encompasses complex Moroccan social relations is beside the point. What she helps us understand is that proverbs are a valuable tool through which we can look into the latent social ethos of this group of people.

Consider the following, Writing Exercise 5.3 from Appendix B:

WRITING EXERCISE 5.3

List five proverbs, in order of importance, that you have heard repeatedly in your family, extended community, and/or society and that have had an impact on your life. Describe briefly the context in which each of them was used. Select the one most important to you and explain how it influenced your thought, belief, and behavior.

My example, Writing Sample 5.3, provides five proverbs from my childhood that represent my familial and Korean societal values.

Rituals and Celebrations

Like routines, rituals and celebrations are also repetitive in nature although they do not always adhere to rigid schedules and time cycles. Rituals and celebrations include both formal and informal and happy and sad occasions. They are associated with personal events such as birth, a rite of passage, marriage, and death; with familial events such as birthday parties, New Year's family reunions, and harvest celebrations; and with social events such as a presidential inauguration, Memorial Day parade, religious ceremonies, and a graduation ceremony. Some are more symbolic, official, ceremonial, or conventional than others.

Through participation in rituals, people gain community knowledge and become socialized. Foltz and Griffin (1996) write about their transformation process during their study of rituals. They began an ethnographic study with a "small group of Witches," initially as participant observers and later as observant participants, and discovered that "the power of ritual had much to do with these changes in [their] inner landscape" (p. 324). They continue, "Turner (1967) saw ritual as a passage where genuine transformations of character and social relationships may occur." For this reason, inventorying personal, familial, and social rituals in which you have participated will illuminate how your character and social relationships have been shaped by such rituals.

Consider the following, Writing Exercise 5.4 from Appendix B, to record and reflect on rituals you have been part of in your life.

WRITING EXERCISE 5.4

List five personal, familial, or social rituals, in order of importance, in which you have participated. Briefly describe the context of each ritual. Select the most important one and describe it in detail in terms of who, when, where, what, and how. Explain why it is important in your life.

My examples are provided in Writing Sample 5.4.

Mentors

Mentors are "wise and trusted guide[s] and advisor[s]" or "teacher[s] or trusted counselor[s]" according to Wordnet Search 3.0 (Princeton University, 2006). The term is often used in vocational or instructional settings. However, in this book I suggest that the term be used broadly to include anyone—whether older or younger than you—from whom you have learned new knowledge, skills, principles, wisdom, or perspectives that have made an impact on your life. Although the mentor-mentee relationship alludes to a hierarchical relationship between a master and an apprentice, it need not preclude horizontal relationships because, as Mead (1978) observed, socialization can happen in all directions—from the older to the younger in "postfigurative culture," from the younger to the older in "prefigurative culture," and within the same generation in "cofigurative culture." Cultural acquisition and transmission often take place between mentors and mentees because mentors intentionally or unintentionally invite mentees to share their knowledge, skills, and perspective from their cultural groups. With or without intention, mentors make durable impressions on mentees through their enduring relationships.

Marian Wright Edelman (1999), civil rights activist and attorney and the founder of Children's Defense Fund, wrote a memoir, *Lanterns*, with the theme of mentors. She includes her father, a personal friend, ministers, and teachers as her mentors:

> Three Black men, my daddy, Morehouse College president Benjamin E. Mays, and his mentee Dr. Martin Luther King, Jr., and three White men, Morehouse College board chair Charles E. Merrill, Jr., my college professor, historian Howard Zinn, and former Yale Chaplain, William Sloane Coffin, Jr., played pivotal roles at key points in my life. What they all had in common was their respectful treatment of me as an important, thinking individual human being. They expressed no sense of limits on my potential or on who they thought I could become, and they engaged me as a fellow wayfarer and struggler. They saw me inside and not just outside and affirmed the strengths I had *because* I was blessed to be born a Black girl child." (p. xvii)

Her metaphor "lanterns" for mentors is appropriate because they illuminate paths of uncertainty.

Despite their positive influences on her, Edelman could not help but acknowledging that her mentors were all men. This male dominance rings true to many women in the professions, especially in academia, according to Rushing (2006). In her posthumously published study of "over 200 women and their life transformation," this feminist scholar juxtaposes experiences of others with her own and analyzes how the academic culture of mentoring has shaped and socialized them into the masculine framework of profession. My own academic mentors were all men except for one; yet the list of my lifelong mentors (Writing Sample 5.5 in Appendix B) shows a different picture.

Follow Writing Exercise 5.5 to reflect on and write about your mentors.

WRITING EXERCISE 5.5

List five mentors, in order of importance, who have made significant impacts on your life and briefly describe who each person is. Select one and explain how this person has influenced you.

Cultural Artifacts

Cultural artifacts are objects produced by members of the society that explicitly or implicitly manifest societal norms and values. As the physical foundation of a society, artifacts are ubiquitous in all levels and periods of culture. Yet they are often misconstrued as antiquated items displayed in museums, representing only traditional societies. This overdrawn association between artifacts and antiquity often misleads people to overlook their own backyards in searching for the material evidence of omnipresent culture in their lives. For example, a soccer ball, whether it is made of leather, rubber, or soda can, is a pivotal artifact of soccer players' culture, indispensable to its very existence. My soccer player son would definitely agree with this statement.

According to cognitive anthropologists, cultural artifacts are not culture per se, only a manifestation; others consider "material culture" a vital aspect of culture (Erickson, 2004). Whichever perspective one adopts, it cannot be denied that artifacts are visible everywhere. They have utility or ceremonial value, incorporated into the life of people. By identifying artifacts important to your life (Writing Exercise 5.6 in Appendix B), you will be able to examine what constitutes your primary culture.

WRITING EXERCISE 5.6

List five artifacts, in order of importance, that represent your culture and briefly describe what each artifact represents. Select one and expound on the cultural meaning of this article to your life.

My list of artifacts is provided in Writing Sample 5.6.

Visualizing Self

"One picture is worth a thousand words." This proverb implies that a visual image can convey a message more efficiently and powerfully than a series of words. The power of visualization as a communication tool is enhanced by the simplicity and succinctness of a visual image into which complex texts are condensed and captured.

Condensation and reduction take place when ethnographers turn voluminous data into an ethno(people)-graphy(image) of an event such as a high school reunion (Ikeda, 1998), a people group such as a high school class (Ortner, 2003), an organization such as a community college (Shaw, Valadez, & Rhoads, 1999), a modern community such as a semirural U.S. town and its high school (Chang, 1992a), and a traditional community such as a Kwakiutl village (Wolcott, 2003a). However complex the culture seems, ethnographers tried to capture it into something comprehensible and manageable for future analysis and interpretation.

Visualization strategies such as kinship diagrams and free drawing apply the principle of condensation and reduction to visual representation. They intend to help stir your memories and organize loosened memory fragments into a visual structure such as a diagram, chart, or drawing. Once bits of data are shaped in a simplified visual image, you can then "unpack" the image for readers in writing. In this writing, you contextualize the image with necessary background information. Although you are not yet at the stage of full-fledged cultural interpretation, visualization activities mix the collection of your personal memory data through self-reflection and self-introspection with cultural analysis and interpretation through organization and explanation.

Kinship Diagram

The family, whether nuclear or extended, constitutes the most intimate and basic kinship system through which members are en-culturated. A nuclear family is made up of one or two generations of immediate relatives created by marriage (or other union) and/or birth (or adoption). Traditionally a nuclear family includes a couple or a couple with children, yet the changing family structure calls for redefinition of a nuclear family. An extended family consists of more than two generations of relatives or multiple married siblings, with their immediate families, residing in the same household. As related families extend further, their kinship structure becomes more complex. Whichever composition it may be, the family has a prominent presence in the lives of many of my undergraduate and graduate students as their "cultural autobiography" (Chang, 1999)—an assignment required in my "multicultural education" courses—indicates.

Provided that family, however it is defined, plays an important role in shaping your culture, charting your family relationship will shed light on your intimate social network. A kinship diagram visualizes the family relationships that you have with others through birth, adoption, marriage, or other forms of union. The chart diagram identifies the different relationships by various symbols and lines. Many ethnographers, especially those who have studied traditional societies, have collected genealogies as part of their ethnographic fieldwork (deRoche, 2007). Although examples of ethnographies including kinship diagrams are too numerous to list here, one example may illustrate the importance of such a practice: Chagnon (1968), who conducted a classic (and also controversial) study of the Yanomamö (a native people of southern Venezuela), devoted a whole chapter of his ethnography to the discussion of the kinship-based structure in this society.

Given the importance of kinship to the culture and the methodological merit of kinship diagramming, charting family relations gives a good start to a data collection of your personal memory. The use of "kin-gram"—a term coined by shortening the traditional anthropological term "kinship diagram" to convey a modified strategy from anthropological variations—will facilitate this process of data collection. For this strategy, I have adopted conventional symbols used by anthropologists like Keesing (1976, p. 241), Bates and Fratkin (2003, p. 282), and Peoples and Bailey (2003, p. 190). They include symbols representing spouse, sibling, and parent-child relationships between the living and the deceased. These symbols, however, are not sufficient to document modern variations of family structures diverged from "traditional" families. Therefore, I here add new symbols to reflect modern-day varieties resulting from adoption, divorce, unmarried partnership, and same-sex union. Conventional and new symbols are shown in Figure 5.1.

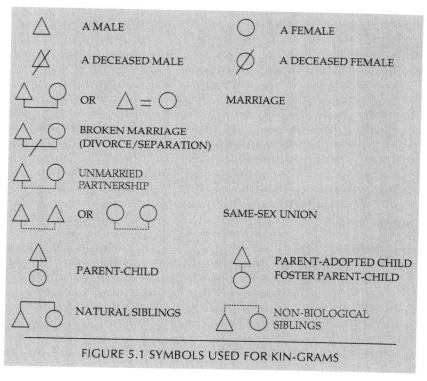

FIGURE 5.1 SYMBOLS USED FOR KIN-GRAMS

Figure 5.2 illustrates my kinship relationships. I here include four generations on my side and three generations on my husband's side whom I got to know personally. I do not include kin on either side with whom I have not had personal contacts or whose impact on me is not significant.

After looking at my kin-gram, you may wonder, "What in the world does the kin-gram say about her family?" This question correctly points out the lack of context that this visualization of kinship structure presents. A subsequent writing exercise will add a contextual body to the skeletal image of my family. In the description of your kinship, you may add as many details as you want to describe individual members, overall family structure, and the sociocultural context of your family. Writing Sample 5.7 in Appendix B describes my kinship structure in writing.

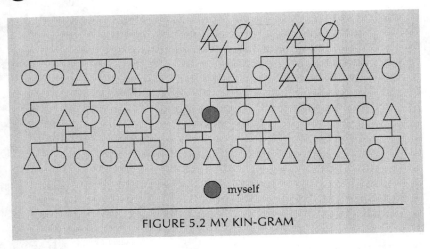

FIGURE 5.2 MY KIN-GRAM

Using the symbols provided in Figure 5.1, I suggest you complete the following, Writing Exercise 5.7:

WRITING EXERCISE 5.7

Create your kin-gram, including all or some key kin who have meaningfully contributed to the shaping of your life. Your kin-gram does not have to include everyone in your family tree. Describe your family on the basis of this kin-gram. Add details about individuals included in it.

Free Drawing

The third visualization strategy is free drawing. Drawing (or doodling) is an excellent prewriting tool to stir up memories. Memory is a vehicle to connect the present to the past. You can draw anything out of your memory: person, object, and place. For this exercise, I encourage you to focus on a memorable space, adopting Wakefield's (1990) suggestion of drawing a favorite room of childhood. In guiding readers to prepare for their spiritual autobiography, this celebrated writer argues that using the "treasure-house of memories" initiates the first step of self-reflective writing. He cites the poet Rainer Maria Rilke's compelling *Letters to a Young Poet*:

[U]se, to express yourself, the things in your environment, the images from your dreams, the objects of your memory. If your daily life seems poor, do not blame it; blame yourself, tell yourself that you are not poet enough to call forth its riches. . . . would you not then still have your childhood, that precious, kingly possession, that treasure-house of memories? (pp. 53–54)

Not everyone may feel that their childhood memories are "precious" and "kingly." Even so, stirring the treasure-house of memories is still extremely useful in the autoethnographic process and is precisely what this visualization strategy intends to accomplish.

This strategy of recalling is particularly wrapped around space. Sack's (1997) notion of human beings as "homo geographicus" also convinces me of the importance of connecting people with their physical environment. According to this geographer, human beings connect themselves with space and place, adjust to them, and, at the same time, effect changes to their natural context. The strong tie between the place of residence and identity is resonated in Taylor's study of women who lived in London at the time of her study (2005). Taylor argues that, regardless of the women's origin, they drew from rich lived experiences of their residence to create a bond with their current place and to develop a place-based identity. The free-drawing strategy promoted in Writing Exercise 5.8 is to help you discover and affirm your "geographic self" and place-based identity. The activity of drawing a series of important places in your lifetime can give you a database with which to interpret the evolution of yourself over time.

Figure 5.3 shows my favorite hiding place of childhood—a shed—where I dreamed a big dream of traveling overseas. This drawing illustrates the connection between who I was and where I was. My description of the shed follows (it is my writing sample for Writing Exercise 5.8).

In the backyard of my childhood home in Korea, two sheds were standing back to back. One stored Korean-style coals for fuel; the other kept miscellaneous junk including "treasures" from my mother's two-year study in the United States before her marriage to my father. Two big black trunks trimmed with shiny "gold" buckles represented the exotic, exciting, and alien land called America. My mom kept in the treasure chests what she had used during her study in America. Her bright-colored flowing dresses

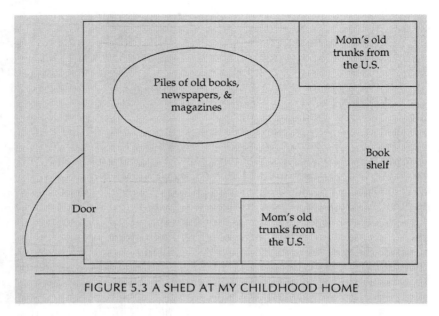

FIGURE 5.3 A SHED AT MY CHILDHOOD HOME

with a tight waist, hats decorated with laces and silk flowers, slim leather belts, white gloves, sparkly jewelry, and high-heel shoes rested inside. They were from the 1950's. None were useable in Korea because a respectable professor would not dream of wearing bright-colored "gaudy" clothes. Other accessories would not match the proper image of a modest middle-aged woman. These treasures were hidden away as if they were heathen temptations.

Musty smells from antiquated books and magazines also permeated the air in this dark shed. Without humidity regulation for many years, the smells seeped into every piece of my mother's old treasures and became a familiar companion to this space. Some children's books and other magazines from the exotic land were strewn in the shelves and on the floor to attest to my previous visit. From time to time I slipped away from my house to sit on the piles of discolored newspapers to read the books, take in the smell of my mom's ancient history, and take out her treasures for dress-ups. America was an alien land; yet, this shed connected me with it with such excitement and comfort. This room is like a wardrobe leading to the mysterious land of Narnia in Lewis' (1978) story. This is a magical space where I dreamt of flying and traveling to other lands.

Slightly diverging from Wakefield's (1990) suggestions, I prefer to open the options of drawing beyond childhood memories, favorite memories, or rooms. For this exercise, you may select a place of significance that is associated with a single memorable event, a ritual, or routine activities. This space may be remembered as a social or a solitary place. It may conjure up a happy or a painful memory. Although you are asked to put down as many details as you remember, your drawing skills and aesthetic presentation are least important. The accuracy of details is also a secondary concern. Rather, through the drawing suggested in the following, Writing Exercise 5.8 of Appendix B, you may discover how the place has shaped your worldview and has affirmed or changed your relationship with others.

WRITING EXERCISE 5.8

Select a place of significance that helped you gain an understanding of yourself and your relationship to others. Draw the place, putting in as many details as possible. You may outline the place or do a realistic drawing. Identify objects and persons in the drawing when necessary. Expand this exercise to additional places. Describe the place and explain why this place is significant to you.

What Else?

Are there more visualization strategies to use when collecting personal memory data? Phifer (2002), a teacher of memoir writing, would answer affirmatively, suggesting a few more "idea-gathering strategies" that trigger visual cues: (1) draw a heart and write in it the names of "people who have been important to you" (pp. 20–21), (2) draw "an overall map" of your childhood home and indicate activities that took place in different locations on it (p. 53), (3) draw a stick figure of self and identify what you wore as a teenager (p. 68), (4) draw a trail and write on it works that you have done (p. 119), and (5) draw a line graph showing the physical, economic, social/cultural, vocational/professional, and spiritual/emotional condition over your lifetime (p. 186). After drawing, I encourage you to provide context information on your drawings.

Wakefield (1990), a novelist and teacher of spiritual autobiography writing, also suggests that spiritual autobiographers draw "a picture of [their] favorite room in the house [they] grew up in" (p. 54) and "a road map" of their life journey including points of significance (p. 94). He argues that this road map will work as "an outline, a reference point, or a starting place" for writing their spiritual autobiography.

In addition to these visualization strategies, mapping a community or a neighborhood where you grew up or currently live or to which you have a special attachment may also be a good beginning. Adding many details and describing the space are still good ideas.

Summary

In this chapter I have suggested various strategies useful in collecting personal memory data. Chronicling refers to a strategy of recalling personal and social events and experiences and giving a chronological structure to them; inventorying is used to list bits of autobiographical information and to rank them by importance; and visualizing organizes personal memories into visual images of charts and figures. Whichever strategies are adopted, you are strongly encouraged to expand them and to create new strategies to meet your research needs. These memory data will be added to other types of data you will collect to create a database for autoethnographic analysis and interpretation.

Collecting Self-Observational and Self-Reflective Data

Autoethnographic data come from your present as well as your past. The previous chapter introduced data collection strategies that tap into what has already happened to you; this chapter presents strategies that help capture your behaviors, thoughts, emotions, and interactions as they occur. Although self-awareness of your research purpose and self-consciousness can affect your data collection, raw data from the present are still useful to the autoethnographic study because, unlike personal memory data, they enable you to preserve vivid details and fresh perspectives.

Autoethnographic data collection from the present is equivalent to ethnographic participant observation in that the researcher in either study collects data from naturally occurring environments while participating in activities. The difference between them is that the data collection field for autoethnography is the researcher's own life whereas ethnographic participant observation focuses on the lives of others (natives of the culture that is studied). In trying to gain cultural perspectives on yourself, you may find strategies of self-observation and self-reflection useful in autobiographical "fieldwork." Self-observation collects factual data of what is happening at the time of research whereas self-reflection gathers introspective data representing your present perspectives. This chapter suggests selected data collection strategies utilizing self-observation and self-reflection.

Self-Observational Data

Self-observational data record your actual behaviors, thoughts, and emotions as they occur in their natural contexts. One way of learning about yourself is observing your own daily or weekly routines for a designated period of time: for example, what you do in solitude or in company of others, what you say, what you feel, what you think, whom you include and exclude in your interactions, where you frequent, and which material objects are necessary in your present life. Typical routines of life illuminate actors' social roles and sociocultural circumstances at a specific time. For example, my daily routines during my college days reflect my life as an unmarried female college student in Korea, which sharply contrasts with those of my present life as a married college professor with children in the United States. Routines of my life today indicate social expectations associated with my present social roles of wife, professor, and parent. Self-observational data from the present, when compared with personal memory data, can reveal changes and continuity in your life over time.

Self-observation can also be applied to explore specific issues in your life. Considering your research purpose, you can identify a certain focus for your self-observation. For example, when I conducted my autoethnography-in-progress on my multicultural experiences, I collected data on my interactions with others of difference over a period of three months whenever they occurred. I recorded my interactions with total strangers whom I had never met before, others of opposition whom I did not like, and acquaintances whom I did not know much about. In my notes, I also added circumstances where such encounters took place. This focused self-observation gave basis to a later analysis of my interaction with others.

Self-observational data collection can be done as a solo activity as you focus on yourself. It can also be stimulated in interactive settings where you actively engage others in your study. This section discusses two different types of self-observation: systematic self-observation as a solitary data collection strategy and interactive self-observation as a collaborative strategy.

Systematic Self-observation

Rodriguez and Ryave (2002) argue that self-observation is a useful data collection technique for qualitative research because it gives access to "covert, elusive, and/or personal experiences like cognitive processes, emotions, motives, concealed actions, omitted actions, and socially restricted activities" (p. 3) and brings to the surface what is "taken-for-granted, habituated, and/or unconscious matter that . . . [is] unavailable for recall" (p. 4). Proposing a systematic and intentional approach to self-observation, they developed the technique of "systematic self-observation" for qualitative studies in which the researcher collects data through self-reporting of research participants who are trained to observe their own behaviors and thoughts. Although the intended use of this technique is with other research subjects than researchers themselves, systematic self-observation can be easily adopted as a data collection strategy for autoethnography.

Self-observation in your daily life takes place casually and informally as you go about your life. For research, however, such self-observation needs to be disciplined by the intentionality of the research process. Planning what to observe and how to observe shapes systematic self-observation. What to observe is determined by your research purpose. How to observe and record needs to be carefully planned out in your research design. For example, you can self-observe and record your behaviors, thoughts, or emotions at certain time intervals or by occurrence; in a narrative format or pre-formatted recording sheets; and immediately when they occur or after you retreat from your action field. All recording methods are useful for different reasons and occasions. You can mix and match, using your researcher judgment and imagination.

Interval or occurrence recording depends on whether observation takes place at pre-set intervals or whenever certain observable thoughts or behaviors occur. The *interval recording* would allow you to observe yourself on a regular basis and chart the flow of your cognitive and behavioral engagements in the course of a set time period—a day, a week, or a month. For example, you may observe yourself every waking hour (e.g., 8 am, 9 am, etc.) for a few separate days or at set times (e.g., 10 am, 2 pm, 6 pm, etc.) daily for a month. With a self-observation schedule carefully planned to meet research goals, you can gain valuable information on the *patterns* of your cognitive engagements, individual behaviors, or interactions with others.

On the other hand, *occurrence recording* intends to produce data on *frequency* of your thoughts or behaviors over a certain period of time. For example, you can record certain types of behaviors whenever you are engaged in them. You can add the contextual information to each occurrence such as how long it lasted, who was present, and what the physical environment was like. Table 6.1 shows an example of occurrence recording of my self-observation on the topic of my people interaction on one day. When such data collection is repeated over a certain period of time, I will be able to look for my interaction patterns with different people at different locations.

TABLE 6.1 AN EXAMPLE OF "OCCURRENCE RECORDING" OF MY SELF-OBSERVATION

Topic: *people I interact with throughout the day and my activities*		**Date:** *3/28/06 (Tuesday): during my sabbatical year*	
Time	Persons in Interaction	Engaged Activities	Location
AM: 6:30–7	daughter	making breakfast for her	home
AM: 8:40–9	son	waking him up	home
AM: 9:15–9:30	husband	talking about today's logistics	home
AM: 10:30–11:30	department's faculty colleague	meeting on grant writing	my school
AM: 11:30–12:10	university staff	meeting on grant writing	my school
PM: 1:15–4:10	instructor and classmates in a painting class	painting and getting comments from the instructor; brief chatting with classmates	my painting class
PM: 5:15–6	son	talk about school	home
PM: 6–6:05	husband	talk about picking up our daughter	home
PM: 6:10–6:30	son & daughter	talk about a party for string players from their youth orchestra	home
PM: 7–8:30	children's teachers and other parents	talk about the children's prospective music trip; chatting with other parents	children's school
PM: 10:20–10:30	son	admonishing for lounging around	home
PM: 11:40–12	husband	talking about kids and grading	home

Self-observation can also be recorded in a narrative format or a pre-structured recording form. Narrative recording allows autoethnographers to describe in detail their observation in a free format. Flexibility of length and format is less likely to inhibit recording, which is the strength of this recording method. On the other hand, a structured, pre-formatted recording facilitates speedy recording and data analysis. By utilizing pre-established codes (e.g., 1=interaction with immediate members; 2=interaction with extended family members; 3=interaction with professional colleagues, etc.), you can turn such standard self-observational data into quantitative data. Table 6.1 illustrates a hybrid model that adapts a structured recording format to accommodate narrative comments.

Self-observation recording can also vary in terms of immediacy. On-site recording refers to immediate recording of thoughts and behaviors that have just occurred or are presently unfolding. This on-site recording is likely to capture immediate emotion, provide a less tampered-with perspective, and record vivid memories of what you just observed. The downside of this method is that your flow of thoughts can be disrupted, and your self-awareness can alter the natural course of activity, which can "taint" data. The benefits and shortcomings of retrospective recording are reversed. When you wait to retreat from your field to record your self-observation, a less-fresh memory is traded for a natural flow of occurrence. As long as the lapse between recording and occurrences of thoughts or behaviors is not great, retrospective recording is useful for autoethnography as well. The ethnographers' disciplined practice of retiring from fieldwork occasionally to record their participant observation will work well for retrospective self-observation. Follow Writing Exercise 6.1 in Appendix C to practice self-observation:

WRITING EXERCISE 6.1

Select a specific behavioral or cognitive topic on which you want to observe yourself. Select a manageable time frame for your self-observation and identify a recording method (narrative, structured format, or hybrid). Conduct systematic self-observation and record your observation including context information such as time, duration, location, people, occasion, and mood.

Table 6.1 is a writing sample for this exercise.

Interactive Self-observation

Interactive self-observation offers another possibility of self-observation by intentionally creating interactions with others in a group setting. One such purposeful group can be a focus group made up of people who share a similar interest or experience with you. Focus groups, synonymous with "group interviews," allow ethnographers to conduct participant observation and interview concurrently by "listening to people and learning from them," according to Madriz (2003, pp. 363–364). This method is used frequently by some circles of qualitative researchers and ethnographers (Bryant, 2007; Kitzinger, 1999; Merton, 1999). Focusing on the shared experience as your research topic, you can co-participate in group discussions. As this collaborative engagement stirs your thought processes, you will be able to observe and record your cognitive, behavioral, and emotional state regarding this topic and your interactions with others of similarity. Rodriguez and Ryave (2002) uses Ellis's term "interactive introspection" to describe the process in which the researchers and the others interview each other "as equals who try to help one another relive and describe their recollection of emotional experiences" (p. 7).

Another type of interactive self-observation can take place when you study others on the topic in which you have a personal interest. This type of interactive self-observation is different from other social science studies merely inspired by the researcher's personal interest without any further consequence on the study. Instead, in this type of interactive self-observation you collect data on others but you enter your perspectives in data analysis by comparing your experiences with others'. Rushing's *Erotic Mentoring* (2006) exemplifies this approach. In this book, she draws a parallel between her experiences and those of over 200 female professionals in male-dominant academia. With a feminist perspective she analyzes gender-based oppression, subjugation, liberation, and transformation, interweaving her story with others. Berger's (2007) autoethnographic writing is based on her ethnographic study of a Messianic Jewish congregation. As she collected data on others, she was pulled into self-observation and self-reflection on her Jewish identity, which she documents in her writing. In both Rushing's and Berger's cases, their self-reflection was recorded as they observed and interviewed others. Their self-reflection entered their autoethnographic writing.

Conduct interactive self-observation as instructed in the following, Writing Exercise 6.2 in Appendix C:

WRITING EXERCISE 6.2

Form a group of two to four people who share similar experiences with you that you want to investigate further. Meet regularly to discuss your experiences. Take notes of your exchanges. Compare and contrast your experiences with theirs. Reflect on how others' contributions to the discussion stimulate your recall of the experiences.

A writing sample for this exercise is provided in Appendix C.

Self-Reflective Data

Self-reflective data result from introspection, self-analysis, and self-evaluation of who you are and what you are. Self-reflection sometimes accompanies self-observation. Therefore, keeping a field journal helps you capture self-reflective data while collecting self-observational data. Self-reflection can also be intentionally and purposefully guided by the research process. For example, the writing exercises suggested here are intended to evoke self-reflection on broad topics such as self-identity, values, preferences, and the relationship with others. More specific topics relevant to your study should be included in self-reflective data.

Field Journal

Ethnographic field journals are used to record researchers' private and personal thoughts and feelings pertaining to their research processes. They are kept separately from field notes that record more objective data from the field. Malinowski's (1967) field diary re-presents a typical field journal, in which he kept his inner, private feelings about informants, sometimes displeasure, and fieldwork. Revealing such secrets was not common in his days, and his diary was not published until 1967, after his death. Nowadays, reflections from the field are often candidly shared in public and even published in professional journals.

In reality, it is difficult to keep "subjective" feelings and "objective" facts completely separate from each other because, while keeping field notes, ethnographers invariably apply their "subjective" judgment and interpretation and, while recording their emotions, they may document situations objectively. Especially in more contemporary ethnographic fieldwork that challenges the dichotomy between subjectivity and objectivity, the division becomes more blurred. Acknowledging the artificiality of this division, some ethnographers allow their data to blend these two components. Crapanzano's *Tuhami* (1980) is an example, in which the ethnographer's representation of a Moroccan informant's visions and dreams blends into the informant's subjective voice. In a case such as this, the rigorous practice of separating subjective data from objective data is almost a moot point.

Although I recognize the difficulty of separating descriptive (objective) data from interpretive (subjective) data, I find that a field journal is a useful vehicle for keeping ethnographic thoughts running during fieldwork. Autoethnographers could benefit from this practice of field journaling as they record reflections on self and the research process. Since autoethnography is a highly self-reflective and introspective process, unless there is a methodical way of keeping a distance from this process, you can easily fall into self-absorption. This meta-cognitive activity of field journaling can provide purposeful and healthy interruptions during fieldwork to help you move into and out of the self-reflective state.

Personal Values and Preference

Culture shapes individuals' "standards for perceiving, evaluating, believing, and doing" (Goodenough, 1981, p. 78). Cultural standards are, in turn, reflected in what you value. Defined as "a principle, standard, or quality considered worthwhile or desirable" (*The American Heritage Dictionary of the English Language*, 2000), cultural values are what you are encouraged to strive for and are encoded in moral standards by which your behaviors and thoughts are publicly and privately sanctioned. Cultural values are manifested in personal preference: liking and disliking of people with whom you socialize, activities you engage in, and materials you possess. Provided that personal values and preference do not rise from a sociocultural vacuum, the analysis of personal values and preference opens the possibility of understanding social ethos. In autoethnographic study, therefore, the analysis of personal values and preference is very useful.

Yet a challenge to such study lies in the fact that values are not always strictly applied or articulated in people's daily lives. Therefore, data on personal values and preference cannot be easily collected by observing behaviors or passing thoughts; rather they come through in the process of self-analysis. In this sense, this self-reflective data collection crosses boundaries between data collection and data analysis. I hope the following, Writing Exercise 6.3 in Appendix C, evokes self-reflection and self-analysis on this topic and spurs further self-reflection on other topics about you:

WRITING EXERCISE 6.3

List five values, in order of importance, that you consider important in your life. Give a brief definition of each in your own terms. Select the most important one and explain why it is important.

My writing example is provided in Writing Sample 6.3.

Cultural Identity and Cultural Membership

Self-reflection can also be applied to the data collection of your cultural identities and group memberships. The culture-gram, a web-like chart, is a tool that I developed to help people visualize their social selves. By completing the chart, you will be able to see your present self from multiple perspectives, in terms of social roles you play, people groups you belong to, diversity criteria by which you judge yourself, and primary cultural identities that you give to yourself.

The culture-gram (see Figure 6.1) contains different types, sizes, and shades of figures and lines connecting them. The figures are designated for four different types of information, and lines indicate connectivity among figures. All the figures connected by lines indicate they belong together in one category.

As you move your attention inward from the outer edge of the chart to the center, I will explain the purpose of each figure. The rectangles are reserved for categories corresponding to multiple realms of life. In my teaching of multicultural education, I have used diversity dimensions for the rectangles and found them to work well for my students. The diversity dimensions include nationality, race/ethnicity, gender, class, religion, language, profession, multiple intelligences, and personal interests.

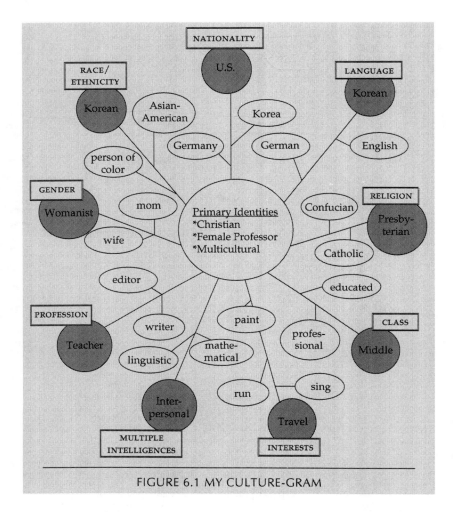

FIGURE 6.1 MY CULTURE-GRAM

You may feel that you do not need all the rectangles, but I suggest that you fill in as many as possible. By stretching your thoughts, you may discover hidden treasures about yourself. Each rectangle is connected to a shaded circle. In each circle, write down one most primary self-identifier of yours in that specific dimension. The self-identifier indicates that you have knowledge, skills, competence, familiarity, *or* emotional attachment to function as a member of this group. This self-identifier is a subjective labeling of yourself, based not on precise measurement but on personal perception and desire. Fill the ovals that are linked to the shaded circle with your secondary self-identifiers in the same dimension. Repeat the same process with other dimensions.

At this point, your culture-gram displays implicitly and explicitly a colorful array of your life experiences, involvements, familiar groups, passions, and cultural competence. Like many of my students who came to this exercise with a belief that they were monocultural or even cultureless, you may be surprised to see how complex and multicultural your life is. Goodenough's (1976) claim that multiculturalism is the normal human experience shines as a truth. In the social milieu where one's culture is often erroneously equated only with race and ethnicity, Goodenough's definition of culture as standards for believing, perceiving, evaluating, and behaving is refreshing. With this definition, it is not possible to deny that all humans are cultural and even multicultural.

The final step of your culture-gramming is filling the center circle with three primary self-identities in the order of importance to you. I selected religious, gender, professional, and cultural identities for the central circle as shown in Figure 6.1. Although not everyone will select his/her religious identity, the gravity of this identity needs to be acknowledged as Kazin considers "religion to be 'the most intimate expression of the human heart, . . . the most secret of personal confessions, where we admit to ourselves alone our fears and our losses, our sense of holy dread and our awe before the unflagging power of a universe. . .'" (cited in Phifer, 2002, p. 125).

Although primary self-identities tend to be enduring and persistent over time, they are not always permanent fixtures in life. Some may remain steady, and others change depending on time, occasion, and context. For example, the essence of my religious and gender identities has remained constant; however, my move to the United States from Korea has affected my racial, ethnic, and linguistic consciousness, which gave rise to my identity recognition as a Korean ethnic, Asian-American, and a U.S.-Korean-German multicultural identity. In the Korean context of ethnic homogeneity, it is conceivable that the lack of personal experiences with different ethnic groups stunted the development of my ethnic self-cognizance.

During 10 years of teaching, I have noticed that my diverse undergraduate and graduate students emphasize different types of identities. My African American students tend to include their racial identity as one of the three primary identities, while White students tend to focus more on nonracial identities. Ethnic, national, or linguistic self-identity is more evident among first-generation immigrant students or international students than native U.S. students. Female students tend to include their gender identity more frequently than male students in their primary identities. This is not based on systematic research, yet the pattern is intriguing and calls for further study.

The culture-gram activity is designed to assist data collection on your present perspective of who you are. However, it is not a simple go-and-gather-facts type of activity. Like other self-reflective data collection strategies, it requires self-reflection, self-evaluation, and self-analysis, which blend data collection with data analysis and interpretation. Writing Exercise 6.4 will guide your self-reflection and self-interpretive process as you chart your self-identities and group memberships in the culture-gram:

WRITING EXERCISE 6.4

Complete the culture-gram (a template is available in Appendix D). Explain three primary identities you selected and your reasons for these selections. Reflect on and write what you have learned about yourself through culture-grammimg.

See Writing Sample 6.4 in Appendix C.

Your culture-gram can also be used to identify others whom you usually distance yourself from, dislike, or oppose for various reasons. Reflect on your "others," such as others of difference or others of opposition, and complete the following, Writing Exercise 6.5 of Appendix C:

WRITING EXERCISE 6.5

 Examine your culture-gram carefully. Make a list of groups of people you are unfamiliar with, dislike, or oppose (among those who are missing from your culture-gram). Select one from your list and write who they are, why you feel the way you do, and where such feelings come from.

Discovering Self Through Other Self-Narrators

The last self-reflective data collection strategy I suggest here is discovering self through other self-narrators. As I argued in Chapter 2, self-narratives are not frozen in a vacuum, severed from others and their sociocultural context. Realistically, self-narratives tell stories about authors as well as their families, neighbors, colleagues, and strangers who are connected to the authors. In stories written by those who have a similar background to yours, you may find a mirror image of yourself. Others are penned by those who come from different situations, sometimes backgrounds oppositional to yours. These self-narrators are teachers who can aid in your self-discovery. You can use other self-narratives as a tool to gather your self-reflective data in two ways.

First, select an excerpt from a self-narrative and write a response to the selected passage. It is useful to select an excerpt that provokes a strong reaction in you, such as agreement or disagreement, approval or rejection, empathy or *schadenfreude* (pleasure taken from someone else's misfortune), applause or criticism. By writing a response to another's life experience and analyzing your reaction to it, you are exploring your beliefs, values, perspectives, and emotions.

The second strategy of self-discovery through other self-narrators involves a compare-and-contrast technique using a Venn diagram. Ideally I suggest that you select one written by an "other of similarity" and another by an "other of difference" to you. By the end of the exercise, you will discover that you are both similar to and different from other self-narrators. This indicates that those who are similar to you by a certain standard are not always similar to you holistically; the case is the same with differences. This discovery is likely to dissipate classification of people on the basis of superficial similarities and differences.

Figure 6.2 demonstrates my example. I selected Tompkins's *A Life in School* (1996) for the reason that the author and I are both female

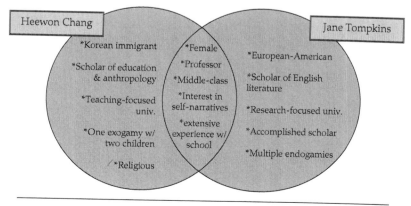

FIGURE 6.2 COMPARISON BETWEEN JANE TOMPKINS AND ME

professors. The Venn diagram displays that we have additional similarities to this professorial role but also significant differences. I might just as well have selected her for the category of others of difference on the basis of our different racial and ethnic identities: she is a European-American White and I am an Asian-American with Korean heritage.

This data collection strategy helps you visually compare yourself with others. Following the instructions of Writing Exercise 6.6 in Appendix C, create a visual comparison between you and a selected self-narrator and translate this visual image into a text. This visual image and text are another example of self-reflective data.

WRITING EXERCISE 6.6

Read a self-narrative and draw a Venn diagram to show similarities and differences between your and the author's life. Select one similarity and one difference from your diagram and describe in detail in what way you and the author are similar to and different from each other. Reflect on and analyze what you have discovered about your culture in the process.

Summary

This chapter presents strategies to help collect self-observational and self-reflective data from your present time, whereas the previous chapter focused on personal memory data. Self-observational data capture your actual behaviors, thoughts, and emotions at the time of data collection; self-reflective data record outcomes of your self-reflection, self-evaluation, and self-analysis. A culture-gram and several writing exercises are suggested to collect a variety of behavioral, cognitive, and emotional data about yourself occurring at the time of study.

Collecting External Data

Given that autoethnography is self-centric in some ways, the primary source of data is *your* past and present. As I discussed in the two previous chapters, personal memory data engender the physical evidence of memory and self-observational and self-reflective data from the present capture the trace of your current perspectives. In either case, data are heavily anchored on *your* "lived experience" and perspectives on "the physical, political, and historical context of that experience." According to Ellis and Flaherty (1992), human subjectivity consists of these two elements of experience and its context, and an investigation of subjectivity tries to connect them. Data from external sources—other individuals, visual artifacts, documents, and literature—provide additional perspectives and contextual information to help you investigate and examine your subjectivity.

Interviews

Interviewing is another staple data collection technique employed in ethnographic fieldwork (Angrosino, 2007; Denzin & Lincoln, 2000; Ellis 2004; Fontana & Frey 2000; Schensul, Schensul, & LeCompte, 1999; Spradley, 1979; Wolcott, 2004). Through interviewing myriad informants, ethnographers gather information unavailable from participant observation. When applied to autoethnography, interviews with others fulfill a different purpose: they provide external data that give contextual information to confirm, complement, or reject introspectively generated data.

A Variety of Interview Techniques

Interviews are used broadly as a qualitative data collection method in social science research. A wide variety of techniques fall within the continuum of individual and group, structured and unstructured, formal and informal, and direct and indirect interviews. Each technique has advantages and shortcomings. The most commonly used type "involves individual, face-to-face, verbal interchange," but other types such as "face-to-face group interchange, mailed or self-administered questionnaires, and telephone surveys" are also readily employed (Fontana & Frey, 2000, p. 645). With easy access to the Internet, emails, online questionnaire surveys, computer-assisted interviews, and online chats are added to this mix. Regardless of the popularity of certain types, you need to select external data collection strategies according to your research needs and circumstances.

An individual interview is conducted with a single individual at a time, whereas a group interview refers to "the systematic questioning of several individuals simultaneously in a formal or informal setting" (Fontana & Frey, 2000, p. 651). Individual interviews are commonly used in ethnographic fieldwork. A separate encounter with each interviewee, in the absence of others, makes it easier for you to preserve confidentiality of information and for the interviewee to become freer from peer pressure. On the other hand, group interviews have a benefit of generating interactions among participants, which can stimulate information flow. A variation of the group interview is a focus group in which specific topics are explored as a group. Bryant (2007) considers group interaction as "a central feature of [the] focus group" and argues, "Because of this interaction, focus groups enable researchers to explore group norms and attitudes, making them valuable in many cross-cultural situations" (p. 116). Group norms and attitudes may be articulated in group exchange. When they are not expressed explicitly, you are given an opportunity to observe as they are quietly played out in the group dynamics.

Structured interviews utilize an interview protocol that contains planned questions in order to avoid digression from your data collection plan. In contrast, unstructured interviews allow flexibility in questioning and responding. Your first question may be planned, but using your research focus as a general guide, you formulate follow-up questions on the basis of interviewee responses during the interview. Since unstructured interviews rely on your quick thinking on the spot, your comfort level with such spontaneity will affect interview quality. Whereas the locus of control is you in structured interviews, power is shared between you and interviewees in unstructured interviews. Structured interviews also tend to take place in prearranged formal settings, and informal conversational settings match unstructured interviews. Both open-ended and close-ended questions can be used in any of the aforementioned interview settings; however, open-ended questions prevail in less-structured interviews, particularly in ethnographic interviews.

Other possibilities are direct or indirect interviews. Direct interviews seek face-to-face exchanges between interviewers and interviewees. Since they can see each other's nonverbal cues during the interview, this format enables them to reap more information than simply what is uttered. On the other hand, face-to-face interviews can discourage them from delving into private, too sensitive, or uncomfortable topics. Direct interviews usually cost more time and money for travels to interview sites than indirect interviews that can be conducted through multiple media, such as phone, email, letter, questionnaire, and Internet. Indirect interviews solve a problem of distance or schedule conflict between interviewers and interviewees. Yet this type of interview takes away the personal and face-to-face advantages.

Ethnographic interviews generally begin with "grand-tour" questions in casual conversational settings and progress to "mini-tour" questions seeking more detailed and focused information (Spradley, 1979). The grand-tour questions are usually general, descriptive, and open-ended. An example of a grand-tour question I used during my U.S. adolescent study (Chang, 1992a) is "Could you tell me about what you do in summer?" "Broad-stroke" questions such as this enable interviewers to safely explore the territory of unfamiliar topics or stranger interviewees. From responses to grand-tour questions, more specific, "mini-tour" questions are spontaneously or methodically derived. For example, when my interviewee responded that he usually works during the summer, I asked him to tell me more about the job he did in the previous summer. Mini-tour questions can still be open-ended and unstructured, but are more specific and focused.

Interviews for Autoethnography

The interview is not commonly associated with autoethnography because this research method focuses primarily on one's own life, while interviews are usually used to draw out life experiences from other people. Therefore, you would not think of the interview first when looking for data collection strategies for your autoethnography. Despite this perception, interviews with others are still useful for this research method for various reasons: to stimulate your memory, to fill in gaps in information, to gather new information about you and other relevant topics, to validate your personal data, and to gain others' perspectives on you.

Your selection of interview formats and question types should depend on your research goals. You can conduct direct or indirect interviews with your family members, friends, colleagues, and strangers. Your familiarity with some interviewees can be both blessing and bliss. Established rapport and the interviewees' knowledge of you help you get to the core of business quickly and more deeply. At the same time, when the topic is about you, your presence may inhibit honest exchanges during interview sessions. To avoid unnecessary alteration of information and ensure interviewee anonymity, a third party may be recruited to administer interviews, an email survey, or a questionnaire. Consider the following, Writing Exercise 7.1 from Appendix E, intended to assist you with interviewing. A writing sample to this exercise is provided in Appendix E.

WRITING EXERCISE 7.1

Make a list of grand-tour and mini-tour questions you would like to ask others about yourself, the context of your life, or other topics relevant to your study. Make a list of potential interviewees who are able to answer these questions. Select one interviewee and make a plan for an interview (name, contact information, method of interview, method of recording, and questions to ask). Conduct an interview. Take notes during the interview, and if possible, audiotape your interview. Produce the interview outcome (interview notes and/or transcripts). Make sure the interview result is clearly marked with identifiers for the purpose of recordkeeping (interviewer name, interviewee name, relationship, topic, interview method, time, and location).

Textual Artifacts

Artifacts are material manifestations of culture that illuminate their historical contexts. Muncey (2005) argues that artifact collecting is a valuable data collection technique in the autoethnographic study because "additional evidence is supplied by meaningful artifacts acquired throughout my life . . . to fill some of the gaps left by the snapshots" (p. 2). Some artifacts are text-based and others nontextual. Living in a text-oriented society, you find ample textual artifacts that enhance your understanding of self and the context of your life. The textual artifacts include officially produced documents and personal, whether formal or informal, texts written by you or about you or your cultural contexts.

Official Documents

Official documents validate significant moments of your life. Although the variety of such documents is too great to name all, they include diplomas, official letters, "certificates, conscription papers, employment contracts, deeds, [and] announcements" (Phifer, 2002, p. 78). Official documents are often produced by social institutions, national or local, which shape and control the social context of your life. Through these official documents, your relations to these organizations are publicly pronounced and, in turn, social norms and standards you abide by are implicated. For example, award certificates define positive behaviors by social standards; police records show the opposite.

Other Textual Artifacts

In addition to official documents, textual artifacts concerning you or authored by you are also useful autoethnographic data. Newspaper articles, bulletins, concert programs, and write-ups about you or your surroundings are only a few examples from the vast range of such documents. Personally produced texts, however, are particularly invaluable to your study because they preserve thoughts, emotions, and perspectives at the time of recording, untainted by your present research agenda. Personal letters, essays, poems, and travel journals from the past are a few examples among many utilized by authors of self-narratives. Personal letters were an igniting flame to Edelman's memoir, *Lanterns* (1999). Edelman unintentionally left behind a bundle of personal letters that she had received during her graduate school days when she graduated and moved away from her rental housing. The letters were discovered many decades later in the attic of her old residence and returned to her. These letters sparked her reminiscences, which led to this insightful self-narrative about her lifetime mentors.

Nash (2002) structures his intellectual memoir around writings he had published in the course of his intellectual career as a professor of philosophy. To a scholar, publications are quintessential artifacts. Therefore, it is appropriate that his published writings play a pivotal role in revealing the evolution of his values and perspectives from different stages of life as a graduate student, a young scholar, an accomplished author, a mature professor.

Another type of self-produced text that Tillman-Healy (1996) uses for her autoethnography is a poem she wrote earlier in her life that expresses her sense of desperation about her bulimic behaviors at the time. On this topic of her lifelong struggle, the poem is positioned appropriately to attest to the historicity of the affliction in her life.

The travel account is a classic example of self-produced writing. Some travel accounts written by missionaries (Olson, 1993) and colonialists such as Christopher Columbus (Mackie, 1891) introduce to their contemporaries exotic others whom they encountered during their travels. Neumann (1992) suggests a different use of travel accounts, namely to look inward at self. He states, "The moments of travel provide a context for entering into other levels of being and belonging to the world that activate latent or potential dimensions of self" (p. 184). Therefore, self-introspection recorded in travel accounts often benefits autoethnographic investigation of self.

The following, Writing Exercise 7.2 from Appendix E, is intended to assist you in collecting textual artifacts, whether they are official documents, your writing, or written texts about you.

WRITING EXERCISE 7.2

Make a list of textual artifacts that you are interested in collecting. For each item identify artifact type, the time and context of its production, access (possible location, contact person, etc.), and data collection date. Select one item and locate the artifact. Describe the artifact and explain what it is for and why it is important to your life.

See Appendix E for my writing sample.

Other Artifacts

Written texts concerning you are limited in telling the full truth about a person, place, or context because they are simply incomplete, lost, or partial. Therefore, other artifacts can be sought out to fill the gaps left by insufficient textual data. The archaic image of "artifacts" associated with dark corridors of museums may cause you to wonder if there is any "museum piece" in your life that is worthy of your attention. For autoethnographic research, artifacts refer to any physical representations of your life. These are ordinary nontextual artifacts that occupy your space, telling stories about your past and present. Photographs, trinkets in your memory box, memorabilia, family heirlooms, souvenirs, video tapes, CD collections, and innumerable other objects are artifacts that you should not ignore as valuable autoethnographic data.

Photographs and Video Images

Visual data complement textual data and sometimes supersede the benefit of textual data because visual data make long-term impressions on viewers. Taylor and Bogdan (1984) write, "The camera is becoming an increasingly popular research tool in the social sciences. . . . Just as a tape recorder can aid in recording data, film and videotape equipment can capture details that would otherwise be forgotten or go unnoticed" (p. 118). Since this passage was written, in the 1980s, imaging devices such as videocameras, digital cameras, and even photo-cell phones have become more advanced and easily accessible. As a result, visual images of yourself and your life context can be readily produced and stored. Some significant experiences are reproduced in your imagination when you review personal photographs and watch videos from your past. What are captured in images are not only persons, objects, and places, but also the invisible social context and personal memories that these images trigger.

Harper (2000) used photography for a qualitative sociological study of Italian city life. He argues, "Photographs document several levels of social life" (p. 721). The photographs record such "mundane information as how many vehicles of what types share the Italian streets at a certain time of day . . . suggest some of the jockeying that regulates a complex mix of human interaction mediated by machines . . . [and] offer evidence of normative behavior" when carefully read "with the help of a cultural insider." His statement implies that one can gather visible data through observation, inferential data through logical reasoning, and cultural data through interpretation from the photographs. These three activities of observation, reasoning, and interpretation can be applied to the broad autoethnographic analysis and interpretation of visual images.

Consider the following, Writing Exercise 7.3 from Appendix E, to collect nontextual artifacts from your life and write about them.

WRITING EXERCISE 7.3

Make a list of categories of nontextual artifacts that you plan to collect for your study. Make the categories broad enough, but not so broad as to be unmanageable. For example, you'll want to list a category as "photos from high school" instead of "photos." Collect artifacts that fit the category. Sort your artifacts into subcategories. Describe briefly the artifacts in one subcategory (type, time and location of its production, others represented by the artifacts, etc.) and write your reflection on the significance of these objects in your life.

See Writing Sample 7.3 in Appendix E.

Literature

In Chapter 4, I mentioned that literature is a useful resource when searching for researchable topics, theoretical perspectives that may frame your study, or other autoethnographic examples written on your topic. At this stage, literature can be consulted for a different reason—to gather information on the sociocultural, "physical, political, and historical" context of your life. Literature serves you as an important source of data that enables you to contextualize your personal story within the public history. In this sense, the literature review gives autoethnography an identity as social science research, intersecting the subjectivity of the inner world with the objectivity of the outer world.

Despite the critical role of literature in autoethnography, the literature review should not dominate the research process. When you gather contextual information on your life, you should remember that literature review is just one of many data collection strategies. Keep your review in appropriate proportion. With your research purpose and topic in mind, a well-crafted literature review plan helps efficient execution of the process.

I suggest that you follow Writing Exercise 7.4 from Appendix E, also printed below, in drafting your literature review plan to streamline your efforts:

WRITING EXERCISE 7.4

On the research topic you selected, make a list of subtopics of which you plan to obtain contextual information. Draft a literature review plan including your main research topic and subtopics. Select one subtopic and conduct a preliminary literature search. If necessary, modify your literature review plan along the way. Take notes during the literature review.

Figure 7.1 is an example of a literature review plan from my study. With the topic of my multicultural transformation, my plan focuses on three cultures with which I have lived experiences: my primary Korean

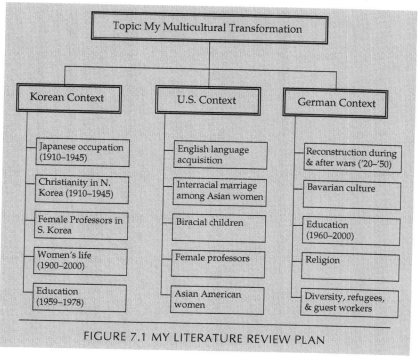

FIGURE 7.1 MY LITERATURE REVIEW PLAN

culture, secondary U.S. culture, and adopted German culture. With a narrowed interest in multicultural issues and the historical contexts that have affected three generations of my family—my parents' (and parents-in-law's), mine (my husband's), and my children's—I select certain time periods and issues on which I concentrate my literature review.

Summary

In this last chapter on data collection, I suggest that data be collected from external sources through interviews with other people, collection of textual and nontextual artifacts, and a literature review. External data provide contextual information, validate or correct your personal data from the past as well as self-observational and self-reflective data from the present, help triangulation with other data sources, fill in gaps left by self-based data, and connect your private story with the outer world.

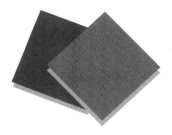

Part III
Turning Data into Autoethnography

As data accumulate, their magnitude and fragmentary randomness can overwhelm you. Although data collection still continues, it is high time to organize the ever-growing data and move forward with steps of turning data into autoethnography. The three chapters in Part III explicate these steps. Chapter 8 introduces data management strategies—labeling, classifying, trimming, and expanding—that help organize and refine data. I argue that data management, collection, and analysis are dynamically interconnected to inform and modify each other. Chapter 9 discusses the critical process of data analysis and interpretation that breathes the spirit of ethnography into auto-ethnography with the emphasis on cultural interpretation. A variety of cultural analysis and interpretation strategies are suggested to help you draw cultural significance from your data. Chapter 10, the final chapter, engages the researcher in the constructive-interpretive process of autoethnographic writing. Writing examples illustrate four different styles: descriptive-realistic, confessional-emotive, analytical-interpretive, and imaginative-creative. In this chapter I encourage you to search for your own style of writing to complete the highly individualized and personalized process of doing autoethnography.

Managing Data

In the previous three chapters I suggested techniques for collecting various autoethnographic data. The data come in the form of fragmented information bits in your field notes, narrative texts, pre-existing documents, still or video images, and many varieties of artifacts. Some data are drawn from your past whereas others are collected at the time of study. Some are personally produced by you and others come from external sources.

As you become more involved in data collection, you may be tempted to throw all data together for later sorting. As the amount of data begins to snowball, however, procrastination with data organization will not only haunt you later but also rob you of two important benefits that timely data management brings. First, periodical organization of data steers the subsequent collection process effectively toward your research goal. While organizing collected data, you can see deficiency (where more data need to be collected), redundancy (where more than sufficient data have already been accumulated), and irrelevancy (where collected data need to be trimmed and discarded) in your data set. This intermediate knowledge of the data set guides your subsequent data collection. Second, clearly labeled and classified data will be readily accessible and identifiable in the later stage of analysis and interpretation. For these reasons, it is advisable to manage data *as they are being collected.*

Data management involves two types of activities: organization and refinement. In this chapter, I suggest a few practical strategies for both activities. Expanding on these, I encourage you to develop your own data organization and refinement system that works for your project.

Data Organization

Data organization is intended to give a logical structure to a mass of collected data by labeling individual data sets and classifying them by categories. A "data set" refers to data bounded by one collection strategy within one set timeframe. For example, a transcript of an interview conducted with one interviewee on a certain date is a data set; so is a writing response you complete for one of the writing exercises suggested in this book. When data are collected, it is recommended that a data set be immediately labeled with a series of simple identifiers by which the data set can be easily located. Labeled data sets become the object of a separate but interrelated activity of classification. They are sorted and grouped by structural and topical categories at the classification stage. These organized data sets eventually become the bases of data analysis and interpretation.

Labeling

A data label provides information about data collection activities as well as the content of the data. The primary—organizational—label quickly reveals something of how the data set was collected: collection time/date, recorder/collector, collection technique, and data source. The secondary—topical—label, which I usually place in parentheses, sheds light on the contextual information or content of the data, expressed in the original timeframe of the data, main actors embedded in the data, topic of the data, and the geographical information on the data. While the primary label helps sort and organize diverse data sets initially, the secondary labeling of data content becomes useful in the later stage of data analysis. For both types of labels, I find the 4-W (when, who, what, where) principle works well.

The "when" information in the primary label reveals the time of data collection and, in the secondary label, the original time when the content of the data took place. For most self-observational and self-reflective data collected at the time of your study, the collection date is when behaviors, thoughts, or events captured in data sets actually happen. Therefore, the historical contexts of data and data collection collapse into one. In the case of memory data, the original timing of the data is different from that of data collection. This means that you have two different contexts to understand when analyzing and interpreting data. The dates in the primary and secondary labels speak volumes about the contexts.

The "who" components in the primary and secondary labels reveal information on (1) who collected and recorded the data and (2) who are the main actors included in your data set, respectively. As an autoethnographer, you are likely to have fulfilled both roles as a collector and a recorder of your personal memory, self-observational, self-reflective data, and possibly interview data. Yet external data such as documents and artifacts are likely to have different authors than you. Depending on who collected which data, you may face different challenges questioning the authenticity and accuracy of data. On the other hand, the second type of "who" element contains a different kind of people information. This label indicates what kinds of others you have included or excluded in your past and present interactions. As I discussed in Chapter 1, our lives are pulled into intentional and unintentional interactions with different others: those who share similar life experiences (*others of similarity*), others who come from backgrounds different from yours or unfamiliar (*others of difference*), and those whose values and experiences you oppose (*others of opposition*). The "who" information in the secondary label gives you a database for the next stage of data analysis and interpretation in which you explore the connectivity between self and others.

The third component, "what," in a primary label tells of data collection types or tools such as interview, self-recollection, and self-observation. This information is useful, considering that certain data types can be more effectively analyzed by one analysis tool than another, although this does not mean that I advocate a one-to-one match between data type and analysis technique. For example, open-ended informal interview transcripts may be qualitatively analyzed through content analysis, whereas activities recorded in a pre-planned self-observation format (see Chapter 6) are better analyzed quantitatively. In addition to this primary "what" information, you are encouraged to add secondary information on the content of the data file. If it is an interview data set, what is the interview about? In the case of self-observation, what was observed? The main topic of the data set corresponds to this "what" component of the secondary label.

The "where" information records primarily where data was collected/recorded and secondarily where the original physical context of the data is. The locality of data collection may stir old memories of yours on the same location. Imagine that your family gather for an annual family reunion at your grandmother's house and reminisce about the time when Grandmother was still living. The location is the same, but the contexts and experiences of your past and present reunion are different. Therefore, the locality component in the primary and the secondary labels sheds different information.

In addition to primary and secondary labeling, I suggest that you paginate each data set if it is textual data. Page numbers will become a compass within each data set during the stage of data analysis. Using any text-creating computer software (e.g., Microsoft Word), you can easily insert labeling information and pagination in a "header."

A labeling header in one of my data files looks like "7-15-06/ Chang/Interview with *Mutti*/Säben (1984 &1990/Chang & Volpert families/family vacation/Säben)." This primary label means that on *July 15, 2006* (when), *Chang* (who) conducted and recorded an *interview* (what) *with Mutti* in *Säben* (where); the secondary label tells that the interview was about the family vacation that the *Chang family and her family* shared (who) in 1984 and 1990 (when) in Säben (where). Primary and secondary information is indeed compacted in this single header. If the header is too long and cumbersome to you, primary labeling information can be easily separated from secondary information to generate simpler labels: "7-15-06/Chang/Interview with Mutti/ Säben" and "1984 &1990/Chang & Volpert family members/family vacation/Säben."

Classifying

Labeled data sets need to be coded and sorted into groups for later analysis (Taylor & Bogdan, 1984). The 4-W (who, when, what, where) criteria again become helpful in this step. The computer becomes a convenient tool for text generation and text analysis. Commercial computer programs[1] exist specifically to assist a qualitative data analysis process. However, here I explain a simple classifying process, using commonly available software such as Excel. Whether you use computer technology for data analysis at all, or no matter which computer program you adopt, one truth remains constant: you are the one who has to decide how to manage, analyze, and interpret data. Neither your decision to use a computer nor your choice of a particular computer program can raise the quality of your study from mediocre to excellent.

Logging labeled data sets is a helpful step in computer-assisted classification. For each file, labeling information should be entered in an Excel sheet as illustrated in Table 8.1.

The data log in the figure contains 11 data sets of various kinds, ranging from interviews to photographic data to self-reflective writing and drawing. The data set number in the first left column indicates the chronology of collection. The next four columns record the 4-W components on data collection from the primary label; the right four columns display information on the content of data from the second-ary label.

Once data are logged, data sets can be easily sorted according to your research needs. All data about Korea (indicated by K), for example, can be sorted and grouped by simply using the "sort" function of Excel by the pertinent column of the log. At this level, data sets can be organized in whichever direction your research calls for. Well-organized data will be much appreciated in the data analysis, interpretation, and writing stages.

Data Refinement

Data refinement is a process of narrowing the focus of data collection and furthering data analysis by trimming redundant and less import-ant data and expanding more relevant and significant data. As data are being collected, it is not possible to determine right away if certain data are more valuable than others and which parts of data will eventually contribute to your analysis. Data organization and initial data analysis will help you discover excess and deficiency in your data.

Initial data analysis begins with coding and sorting. These activ-ities intend to achieve different goals from labeling and classifying data sets. Coding and sorting are used to fracture each data set into smaller bits on the basis of topical commonality and to regroup the data bits into topical categories. For example, after reviewing my collected data, I noticed that my data contain much information about education. So I pulled all bits of data mentioning, implying, and representing education in my life. Education is one topic by which I group a large number of selected data sets. I then decided that I needed to collect no more data on education for the time being and move on to a dif-ferent topic. I also noticed that data regarding my life in the United States did not contain much about my interactions with Koreans. I wondered about it and had to decide if omissions in data reflect my disengagement with the culture or represented something else. My

TABLE 8.1 AN EXAMPLE OF A DATA LOG

Data Set #	Data Collection Strategy (primary labeling)				Data Content (secondary labeling)			
	Date	Collector	Type	Location	Time	People Involved	Source	Place
1	04-9-10	Chang	S/R- culture-gram	U-classroom	2004	self	self	
2	05-9-20	Chang	S/R- kin-gram	U-home	1923–2005	self/KGU-family	self	
3	05-10-15	Chang	S/R drawing	U-home	1976	self/mother	self	K-home/shed
4	05-11-30	Chang	interview	U-conference	1982–1989	self	Dr. W.	U-U of Oregon
5	06-5-10	Chang	interview	K-home	1959–1982	self/K-family	mother	K-family
6	06-5-14	Chang	Vi-photos	K-home	1975–1982	self/ K-family-friends	self/friends/K-family	K
7	06-5-14	Chang	Do-memory book	K-home	1982	self	K-friends	K-church
8	06-5-14	Chang	Do-grade reports	K-home	1972–1982	self	K-teachers	K-middle/HS
9	06-6-30	Chang	S/O-travel journal	O-Istanbul, Turkey	2006	self/U-family/Turkish	self	O-Istanbul Turkey
10	06-7-15	Chang	interview	O-Saeben, Italy	1984–1990	self/G-family	Mutti	G
11	06-7-20	Chang	S/O	G-home	2006	self/G-family	self	G-home

Notes: S/R=self-reflective, Vi=visual, Do=document, S/O=self-observational, U=USA, K=Korea, G=Germany, O=others acknowledgment of this deficiency led me to do self-observation of my contacts with Koreans in my daily routine.

One activity of refinement is "reducing" data. It is an oxymoron that data collection breeds data reduction. This refinement process, commonly incorporated in qualitative as well as ethnographic research, should be contextualized in the distinctiveness of ethnographic and autoethnographic research design. In ethnographic research, you do not follow a rigidly structured data collection plan; you sometimes allow your gut feelings and broadly defined research goals to take a lead in your data collection. This exploratory approach gives your forgotten memories and submerged thoughts a chance to surface during your data collection. In the process, however, many excess data may be collected in one topic while another topic is waiting to be explored. The refinement process occasionally interrupts data collection activities and gives you an opportunity to examine the direction of your data collection.

When data deficiency is noticed in a certain topic, you want to steer and expand your data collection toward filling the gaps. "There are no guidelines in qualitative research for determining how many data are necessary to support a conclusion or interpretation" (Taylor & Bogdan, 1984 p. 139). This is also true of the autoethnographic study. Instead of trying to reach an unknown data quota, it is wise to self-regulate additional data collection as you move along with data analysis. The more you work on the data, the clearer the themes of your study become. The emerging-out-of-the-fog experience will help you also identify which data you need to reduce or expand further.

The Dynamic Process Among Data Collection, Management, and Analysis

The autoethnographic research process is not linear in the sense that one activity leads to the next one and so on until you reach the final destination. Instead, research steps overlap, sometimes returning you to previous steps. One activity informs and modifies another. Figure 8.1 illustrates such a dynamic relationship among data collection, management, and analysis. As you collect data on yourself, you organize your data through labeling and classifying. In the process, you refine your data sets by trimming some and expanding others. This data management facilitates data analysis and interpretation, which I will discuss in the next chapter.

In the same way, the data collection process is often intertwined

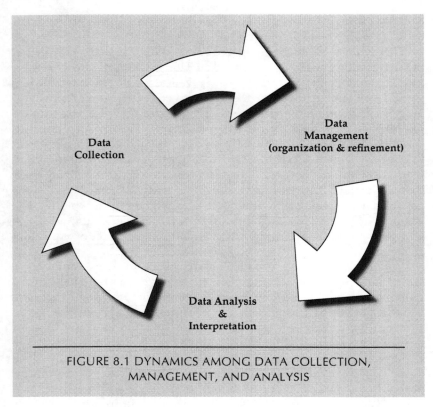

FIGURE 8.1 DYNAMICS AMONG DATA COLLECTION,
MANAGEMENT, AND ANALYSIS

with data analysis and interpretation. Data collection, analysis, and interpretation activities often take place concurrently or inform each other in a cyclical process. For example, when autoethnographers recall past experiences, they do not randomly harvest them. Rather, they select some and discard others according to already-set criteria. Evaluating certain experiences against the criteria is an analytical and interpretive activity. The data collection activities also help researchers examine the validity of their criteria and revise them accordingly. The revised criteria then inform the analysis and interpretation.

Taylor and Bogdan articulate such a dynamic process in a simple sentence: "Data collection and analysis go hand-in-hand" (1984, p. 128). Data management links these two steps.

Summary

Data management is an intermediary link between data collection and data analysis. When data are collected, they need to be labeled and classified so that they can be easily located out of a mass of information. In the process of organization, you will notice gaps and holes as well as excess in your data. You are encouraged to take care of excess and deficiency by trimming and expanding data. As you continue to collect new data and manage collected data, you have already begun data analysis and interpretation. The borderless crossings among activities of data collection, management, and analysis will help you collect more relevant data that are meaningful to your study and your life and prepare you for the steps of data analysis and interpretation.

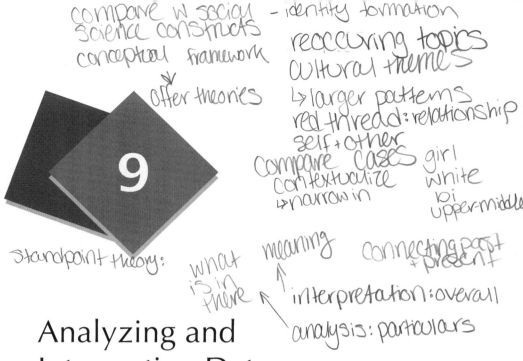

Handwritten annotations:
compare w social science constructs
conceptual framework
offer theories
- identity formation
reoccurring topics
cultural themes
↳ larger patterns
red thread: relationship
self + other
compare cases   girl
contextualize   white
↳ narrow in   bi
    upper-middle
standpoint theory: what is in there   meaning
connecting past + present
interpretation: overall
analysis: particulars

Analyzing and Interpreting Data

whats important   now am I living today as a result of:

By now you will have accumulated a substantial amount of data and be anxious to move onto the "next" step. In an autoethnographic study, moving to the next step, data analysis and interpretation, does not mean abandoning the previous step, data collection, because data collection is likely to continue along with data analysis and interpretation to fill gaps and enrich certain components of data. To assist you with this "next" step, I provide data analysis and interpretation strategies in this chapter. However, a warning is due that no strategy will bring about a quick and easy result in autoethnography. Denzin and Lincoln (1994) articulate the challenge as such: "The processes of analysis, evaluation, and interpretation are neither terminal nor mechanical. They are always emergent, unpredictable, and unfinished" (p. 479).

When analyzing and interpreting autoethnographic data, you need to keep in mind one important point: what makes autoethnography ethnographic is its intent of gaining a cultural understanding. Since self is considered a carrier of culture, intimately connected to others in society, the self's behaviors—verbal and nonverbal—should be interpreted in their cultural context. Therefore, autoethnographic data analysis and interpretation involve shifting your attention back and forth between self and others, the personal and the social context.

Like other ethnographic inquiries, this step in the research process is methodologically nebulous to describe because analysis and interpretation require the researcher's holistic insight, a creative mixing of multiple approaches, and patience with uncertainty. However, careful and skillful interweaving of data collection, analysis, and interpretation will ultimately lead to the production of narratively engaging and culturally meaningful autoethnography.

Data Analysis and Interpretation as the Crux of Ethnography

Data analysis is at the center of research endeavors, whether qualitative or quantitative research. Until you give a meaningful structure to collected data, they may appear to be a "messy" pile of fragmented bits. Data analysis and interpretation are the processes through which the data become a cogent account of observed phenomena. Ethnographers look for cultural themes with which they organize the mess of information.

Cultural data analysis and interpretation are also quintessential to autoethnography because this process transforms bits of autobiographical data into a culturally meaningful and sensible text. Instead of merely describing what happened in your life, you try to explain how fragments of memories may be strung together to explain your cultural tenets and relationship with others in society. In this sense, autoethnographic data analysis and interpretation distinguish their final product from other self-narrative, autobiographical writings that concentrate on storytelling.

Analysis and interpretation enable researchers to shift their focus from merely "scavenging" or "quilting" information bits to actively "transforming" them into a text with culturally meaningful explanations. Some selected segments from raw data are likely to enter your final autoethnography, but not all bits and pieces of data appear in their entirety. When vignettes and excerpts from the data are adopted into the final text, their edges are trimmed and blended into the picture as whole so that they can tightly hang together within the overall structure of cultural analysis and interpretation of self. Therefore, the cliché "Let the data speak for themselves" does not tell the full truth of the ethnographic process. You need data, but you should be the one who gives a culturally meaningful account for data. Data are there to support and illustrate your arguments, but not to stand alone to tell the story. You are expected to review, fracture,

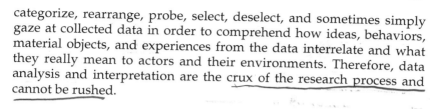
categorize, rearrange, probe, select, deselect, and sometimes simply gaze at collected data in order to comprehend how ideas, behaviors, material objects, and experiences from the data interrelate and what they really mean to actors and their environments. Therefore, data analysis and interpretation are the crux of the research process and cannot be rushed.

Are Analysis and Interpretation Synonymous?

The two terms, data analysis and data interpretation, are often used as a pair. Are they then synonymous? Wolcott (1994) argues that they are not the same although not independent from each other. For conceptual clarity, he chose to explain these in two separate sections of his book, *Transforming Qualitative Data: Description, Analysis, and Interpretation*. He describes data analysis as an activity directed to "the identification of essential features and the systematic description of interrelationships among them—in short, how things work. In terms of stated objectives, analysis also may be employed evaluatively to address questions of why a system is not working or how it might be made to work 'better'" (p. 12). Analysis urges you to stay close to data and "work on" them.

Differing from data analysis, data interpretation focuses on finding cultural meanings beyond the data. Interpretation "involves making sense of the data" (Creswell, 1998, p. 144) and "addresses processual questions of meanings and context. 'How does it all mean?' 'What is to be made of it all?'" (Wolcott, 1994, p. 12). Meanings are not available from the data as ready-made answers; rather they are formulated in a researcher's mind. Hodder (2003) articulates the relationship between meanings and texts as such: ". . . meaning does not reside in a text but in the writing and reading of it. As the text is reread in different contexts, it is given new meanings, often contradictory to each other and always socially embedded. Thus there is no 'original' or 'true' meaning of a text outside specific historical contexts" (p. 156).

The historical contexts that shape meanings of specific texts (data) for insiders (informants or habitants of a culture) are different from those of outsiders (researchers) who try to make sense of data. In a conventional ethnography, insiders and outsiders are different people; therefore, it takes outsiders a considerable number of border-crossing experiences to decipher the cultural meaning of data collected from insiders. In autoethnography the insider and the outsider converge. Namely, you are a generator, collector, and interpreter of data. For this reason, you are familiar with two different contexts: the original context of data and the context of autoethnographic interpretation and writing. During data interpretation, you excavate meanings from two different contexts and wrestle with contradictions and similarities between them.

Analysis and Interpretation as a Balancing Act

So far, a conceptual distinction between analysis and interpretation has been made. In reality, however, data analysis and interpretation are often conducted concurrently and their activities are intertwined. For this reason, strategies of analysis and interpretation presented in this chapter are not strictly separate, although some may be more inclined to analysis and others to interpretation. It is also possible that you make a transition from data analysis to data interpretation, and in the reverse direction, without noticing your cognitive gear-shifting. Thus, analysis and interpretation should be seen not in conflict with each other, but as a balancing act between fracturing and connecting, between zooming in and zooming out, between science and art.

The first balancing act is between fracturing and connecting. In the simplest terms, analysis tends to dissect a data set whereas interpretation urges researchers to connect fractured data. According to Maxwell (2005), fracturing is part of the data analysis called "categorizing" that refers to two main activities—"coding" and "organizing" data. The activity of coding "'fracture[s]'. . . the data and rearrange[s] them into categories that facilitate comparison between things in the same category and that aid in the development of theoretical concepts" and the activity of organizing "the data into broader themes and issues" (p. 96).

Let me use my memory data on a family trip to illustrate the fracturing (coding) element of the categorizing activity. For this particular family reunion, my family of four went on an overnight trip with my parents, one unmarried sister, and two married sisters with their families. My memory data contain descriptions of what happened during the trip and my reflections on the family reunion. As I was reviewing the account of this event, I marked different segments of data with prevalent topics such as parents-daughter relationships, sisterhood, parenting, family conflicts, celebration, meal sharing, and leisure activities. Coding refers to assigning topical identifiers to different segments of the data. Then data segments are grouped by topical code; such groups are again put together into a larger category such as "family dynamics" and "family traditions." The coding and organizing activities of fracturing may seem tedious at times, yet they give a foundation for the connecting activity.

Maxwell (2005) considers "connecting" a part of analytical activities, in which qualitative researchers make "attempts to understand the data . . . in context, using various methods to identify the relationships among the different elements of the [data]" (p. 98). When you classify and connect fragmented data according to themes drawn from your data, you are still doing data analysis because your activity focuses on your data. When you search for connections between your data and sociocultural contexts, you have moved to data interpretation. This transition is absolutely necessary in gaining a comprehensive understanding of your autobiographical data.

The second act of balancing in data analysis and interpretation involves zooming in and out of collected data. The zoom-in approach refers to the "microscopic" analysis of data through which you pay attention to details, probe into small segments at a time, and keep a focus on one data set at a time. This approach enables you to turn your attention to interesting details and their interconnectivity within and between your data sets while keeping blinders on with respect to the big picture and the broader context. Zooming in relates to analytical categorizing and fracturing data mentioned above. Whereas analysis is more likely to direct you to zoom in at one data set at a time, interpretation tends to pull you away from details to hover over the entire data and the context. The zooming-out approach privileges you with a bird's-eye view to the data, which will enable you to see how your own case is related to others, how your case is connected to its context, and how the past has left traces in the present. An ideal data analysis and interpretation process combines the zoom-in and zoom-out approaches. Zooming in elicits "ethnographic details"; zooming out engenders overarching cultural themes (McCurdy, Spradley, & Shandy, 2005, p. 67).

The third type of balancing act considers the different disciplinary orientations stemming from science and art. The scientific orientation of research prescribes transparency, predictability, objectivity, and a systematic approach to research methodology. Although social scientists, including some anthropologists, practice the scientific process of generating and testing hypotheses and formulating generalizable theories, many of them acknowledge that social "science" cannot create a totally objective, value-neutral environment to study. Qualitative researchers, including ethnographers, have accepted the value-laden human reality and the cultural predisposition of researchers. Therefore, they have often allowed nonscientific factors— "the three 'I's'" of "insight, intuition, and impression" (Creswell, 1998, p. 142)—to influence the ethnographic process.

The three "I's" meet with personal creativity and imagination of autoethnographers as well. These nonscientific factors are necessary in the autoethnographic process because a holistic understanding of a cultural case requires a comprehensive approach. In this sense, autoethnography swings away from science. However, I propose that the artistic dimension of autoethnography be "disciplined" so that interpretation is anchored on systematically collected and analyzed data, not merely on personal impressions and reflections. The artistic dimension of data interpretation makes the methodological instruction of this research less mechanical and "unpredictable" (Denzin & Lincoln 1994, p. 479) and "most mysterious" especially to "novice researchers" (Maxwell 2005, p. 95). Considering the science-art contrast, you should keep in mind that strategies presented in this chapter are intended as initial systematic tools to assist data analysis and interpretation and that a "custom-tailored" approach is absolutely necessary in auto-ethnographic data analysis and interpretation.

Start Early

By now you may have collected a *substantial*, but not complete, body of data to "work on." The data are incomplete in the sense that data collection for refinement is likely to continue along with data analysis and interpretation. This implies that data analysis and interpretation do not need to wait until data collection is fully concluded.

Wolcott (2001) suggests that you begin writing early in the ethnographic process, even during the early stage of fieldwork, because it stimulates and facilitates data collection and eventually stimulates cultural analysis and interpretation. Maxwell's (2005) suggestion resonates. He states that "the experienced qualitative researcher begins data analysis immediately after finishing the first interview and observation, continues to analyze the data as long as he or she is working on the research, stopping briefly to write reports and papers" (p. 95). He likens qualitative data analysis to the working of an experienced mountaineer who "begins lunch immediately after finishing breakfast and continues eating lunch as long as he or she is awake, stopping briefly to eat supper" (p. 95). The advice of beginning data analysis early is also given by many other seasoned ethnographers (McCurdy, Spradley, & Shandy, 2005; Taylor & Bogdan, 1984).

In autoethnography, this advice is even more applicable and doable because you enter into a research project with the pre-knowledge of your life. Therefore, you are predisposed to begin connecting data fragments and contextualizing them without having to wait until data collection is advanced. For this reason autoethnographic studies can achieve much more organic transition from data collection to data analysis and interpretation.

How do you begin data analysis and interpretation? For qualitative researchers Maxwell (2005) suggests "reading" textual data and "listening" to oral data as the initial step (p. 96). The suggestion applies as well to autoethnography. At this initial stage, you should review data by segment, as they are collected or classified, as well as holistically. Segmental reading refers to reviewing each data set separately as originally collected or a topical category of data as initially analyzed and rearranged. Holistic reading means reviewing the entire data through with little interruption. Both sectional and holistic reviews open you to a broad understanding of what is in the data, what the data say, and what the data mean.

Analysis and Interpretation Strategies

During the initial reading and listening, you should keep "memos" of your impressions as to repeated topics, emerging themes, salient patterns, and mini and grand categories. You should also code and organize data, which I discussed in Chapter 8. Now you are ready to apply more focused efforts of data analysis and interpretation to your data. Here I suggest 10 strategies[1]: (1) search for recurring topics, themes, and patterns; (2) look for cultural themes; (3) identify exceptional occurrences; (4) analyze inclusion and omission; (5) connect the present with the past; (6) analyze relationships between self and others; (7) compare yourself with other people's cases; (8) contextualize broadly; (9) compare with social science constructs and ideas; and (10) frame with theories. There is no magic to the number 10 or to the order of listing except for the general rule that the earlier ones are more analysis oriented and the later ones are more interpretation oriented. As I have repeated numerous times in this book, researchers should take this list as helpful suggestions, not as a complete tool kit of data analysis and interview.

Search for Recurring Topics

One simple strategy of analysis is identifying recurring topics, themes, or patterns by holistically reviewing the entire data or partially reviewing fractured data bits. Topics refer to specific subjects pertaining to people, places, ideas, or activities. For example, my writing samples for writing exercises (see Appendices B, C, and E) contain several references to the value of education. This is one example of a recurring topic. Topics may become categorical labels with which data may be fractured and organized. When a topic appears frequently in the data, it is likely to signify its importance in your life. Therefore, search for repetition to discover foundational elements of your life.

Look for Cultural Themes

Looking for cultural themes is considered "an important final step in the ethnographic process" (McCurdy, Spradley, & Shandy, 2005, p. 79). A cultural theme is defined as "'a postulate or position, declared or implied, and usually controlling behavior or stimulating activity, which is tacitly approved or openly promoted in a society'" (p. 78). Therefore, a theme describes relationships among various elements. For example, "my family values education" is a theme that dominated my childhood as well as my adult life. Therefore, this theme pops up at many different spots in my autobiographical data. Themes like this are too abundant and palpable in the data to miss after a quick reading of my data. Others such as "My Christian faith is at the root of my sense of justice" are too latent to be easily "excavated." Or the theme such as "Educational credentials are greatly valued in Korean society" cannot be contained in one topical category of data. Rather, as Shank (2002) notes, themes and patterns "seem to cut across various aspects of the data" (p. 129). Therefore, you need to search for them and abstract them from global and holistic reading of data. In that sense, Shank challenges the notion of "emerging" themes that some qualitative researchers casually adopt, citing Morse's (1994) articulation:

> Doing qualitative research is not a passive endeavor. . . theory does not magically emerge from data. . . . Rather, data analysis is a process that requires astute questioning, a relentless search for answers, active observation, and accurate recall. It is a process of piecing together data, of making the invisible obvious, of recognizing the significant from the insignificant, of linking seemingly

unrelated facts logically, of fitting categories one with another, and attributing consequences to antecedents. It is a process of conjecture and verification of correction and modification, of suggestion and defense. It is a creative process of organizing data so that the analytical scheme will appear obvious. (p. 25)

Through the process that Morse describes, researchers identify themes. The themes—main or sub—can frame the final writing of autoethnography.

Identify Exceptional Occurrences

While repetition and recurrence give much information about our lives, not all aspects of our lives follow patterns and routines. As a matter of fact, exceptional events and encounters often change a course of life and make major impacts on life. Many first-time cross-cultural experiences open eyes to new perspectives, cultural standards, people, and environments. After life-changing experiences, people rarely go back to their old selves, but rather move on to a new direction. For this reason, identifying exceptional occurrences in life can provide tremendously useful information on self. You can structure your data analysis and interpretation around these exceptionalities in life.

Analyze Inclusion and Omission

Data analysis and interpretation usually deal with what is included in the data set, namely, what is collected and what the collected data represent. However, we should not forget that what is omitted in the data also sheds valuable light on the data. The absence of data comes from different reasons. On one hand, some elements are simply absent in one's life, thus nothing is there to record in data. On the other hand, omission in data can result from intentional or unintentional exclusion of them in recording. One way of discovering omission in data is through asking a question about omission for each inclusion. For example, when I analyzed my list of professional mentors, I looked for patterns of my mentors—in terms of gender, age, ethnicity, profession, and context of contacts. Most of my professional mentors in life have been males, as was the case with Edelman (1999). Then I asked myself why women were mostly missing in my professional mentoring relationships. I had to ask myself a second question: Were there indeed scarce female mentors in my life, did I accidentally or purposefully leave out female mentors, or did I refuse mentoring relationship with females? Omission in data reveals an autoethnographer's unfamiliarity, ignorance, dislike, disfavor, dissociation, or devaluation of certain phenomena in life. Above all, it may illuminate what is valued and devalued in the society.

Connect the Present with the Past

This history-conscious strategy helps autoethnographers discover how their present thoughts and behaviors are rooted in past events. The seeming cause-effect relationship is never established with certainty in this strategy, although researchers may desire to make a clear connection between the past and the present. For example, I cannot definitely "correlate" my choice of a professorial career with my parents' choices of academic profession and my childhood exposure to their professional lives, although the connection is feasible. Without "scientific" tools to establish correlation, you need to resort to logical reasoning, imagination, and intuition to explain the connection between the present and the past. This connection, albeit an approximation, is a reasonable option to explore in autoethnographic analysis and interpretation.

Analyze Relationships Between Self and Others

Searching for the connectivity between self and others is fundamental to autoethnographic interpretation. Austin (1996) reminds us that "the essence of who we are, what we think, and how we talk is contingent largely on the others we celebrate" (p. 206). The others that Austin refers to here are *others of similarity* as discussed in Chapter 1. This type of others includes those who belong to the same community of practice, share common identities, and/or identify with each other. During data analysis and interpretation, you can ask yourself questions such as "Who are my others of similarity?" "What binds us together?" "What forms the foundation of my bonding with these others of similarity?"

In addition to others of similarity, you can also look for *others of difference* in your life. The others of difference represent communities of practices, sets of values, and identities different from yours or unfamiliar to you. These others often help you see yourself more clearly by contrast. In some occasions you may consider merely different, others irreconcilably oppositional. Reflecting on her ethnographic experience in Morocco, Anderson (2000) perceptively contrasts the Arab's notion of self with her American one: "The Arab's very 'social self' upsets Americans who, although rarely verbalizing it, anticipate a predictable consistency in social interactions, a fixed internal (not external) monitor of right and wrong. The Arab thrives on a 'negotiable' self. . . . In the Arab world one accounts for one's actions to a viewing society; in ours, essentially, to that constant voice within" (p. 104). She figuratively speaks her sense of profound difference between Moroccan self and American self: "We were never meant for marriage." Her sense of difference is not explicated in hostility or dislike. In contrast, "her affection for Morocco and the lingering memory of its beauty" is genuine; yet her perception of difference is real and unequivocal. Anderson's assessment of Moroccans comes close to the borderline between *others of difference* and *others of opposition*.

In my autoethnographic analysis I discovered that Japanese used to be my others of opposition. Having grown up in post-colonial anti-Japanese Korea with parents who were victimized by 36 years of Japanese occupation, I did not have difficulty pronouncing my dislike and ignorance of Japanese and Japanese culture until I confronted my prejudice in my adult life (see my writing sample 6.5 in Appendix C). In my case, others of opposition were initially imagined enemies that later turned into others of difference and eventually others of similarity.

Using the typology of others, you can identify and characterize others included and omitted in the data. Consider the following questions: What kinds of others are included in your data? What is the relationship between yourself and these others? Which types of others are left out of the data? Why are they left out? The analysis of self-other relationships can be extended to other analysis and interpretation strategies such as cross-case comparison and broader contextualization discussed later.

Compare Cases

Comparison is an exercise useful in identifying similarities and differences between two separate cases. In an autoethnographic study, different people, events, or contexts can be drawn from the data. For example, I compared my Korean and German families and wrote about parallels between them in my writing sample 5.7 in Appendix B. Persons can also be objects of comparison, as I illustrated in my comparison with Jane Tompkins in Figure 6.3 in Chapter 6. By comparing my case with someone who belongs to the same community of academic practice, I gained tremendous insight as to commonalities and differences between us and our social contexts. Foster, McAllister, & O'Brien (2005) argue, "What matters is that difference and commonality are consciously addressed, rather than dismissed or minimized throughout the meaning-making process" (p. 9). The strategy of comparison indeed brings "difference and commonality" to your consciousness and further understanding of self.

Contextualize Broadly

Data analysis and interpretation strategies so far have focused more on your personal data. This strategy of contextualization shifts attention to what lies beyond your case, the broadly termed "context." The metaphorical expression of zoom in and zoom out, discussed earlier, illustrates the strategy of contextualizing. Through this strategy, one attempts to explain and interpret certain behaviors and events in connection with the sociocultural, political, economical, religious, historical, ideological, and geographical environment in which they took place and in which data were recorded.

An in-depth understanding of the context, an imperative in cultural interpretation, does not come by narrowing your focus to your autobiographical data only, but rather through external sources such as literature about the context and interviews with others. To make cultural interpretation manageable, you should set a boundary by determining how broadly you want to define the context. In my case, I had to ask myself if I wanted to review the history of contemporary Korea back to 1898 when my grandmother, the matriarch of my household, was born, or if I wanted to focus on a more recent Korea that gave a sociocultural and political context to my life. A similar question can be asked about the geographic boundaries. You will have to decide where to limit your context: your neighborhood, local community, microculture,[2] or nation.

Compare with Social Science Constructs

While the previous strategy of "contextualizing broadly" starts with your case and extends out to the context, this strategy starts outside, particularly in the literature, and moves into the case. It uses social constructs as a window through which autobiographical data are interpreted. Creswell (1998) notes the possibility of applying social constructs in qualitative data interpretation. A social science construct is an abstract or general concept or idea constructed to explain social phenomena. A construct from social science literature can become a conceptual framework for your autoethnographic analysis and inter- pretation. In my autoethnography, I used "multiculturalism" as a social science construct to interpret the cultural evolution in my life.

Frame with Theories

This strategy is similar to the strategy of adopting social science con- structs in that the framework for data analysis and interpretation comes from the literature. The difference between this strategy and the previous one is that the former uses a concept as a framework and this adopts a theory to explain phenomena in autobiographical data. The term "theory" in this strategy does not imply a hard core "tested hypothesis" in a scientific sense. Rather, I use the term casually to refer to a conjecture or postulate that explains a social phenomenon. Theories, therefore, are considered as explaining tools. Although es- tablishing a new theory is not a goal of autoethnography, utilizing an existing theory to explain your case is possible. With this strategy, chosen theories can guide the process of data organization, analysis, and interpretation, and the structure of writing.

Summary

Data collection and interpretation are at the crux of autoethnography. What you search for in the mass of data is indicators that can ex- plain how your life experiences are culturally, not just personally, meaningful and how your experiences can be compared with others' in society. Therefore, in this process you zoom in on the details of your life and zoom out to the broad context. This process also balances two opposing activities of fracturing data and connecting fragments to create a coherent story and cultural explanation. Several data analysis and interpretation strategies suggested in the chapter are intended to assist you with making cultural sense out of the mass of data.

Writing Autoethnography

Autoethnographic writing activities are expected to begin early and to be practiced steadily throughout the research process. You write when recording your personal memories and self-observation during data collection. If you are not writing responses to the writing exercises suggested in Chapters 5 through 7 or other textual data, I imagine that you will be taking notes of your reflections, ideas, and impressions while reviewing data. As you are making progress in data analysis, you may also keep a record of emerging themes.

Now you face a new kind of writing—writing a complete autoethnography. This requires a different frame of mind and new strategies. Your focus needs to shift from sifting through masses of fragmented details to stringing discovered gems together in an intriguing pattern so that the finished product will sound cohesive and interesting. Writing an autoethnography represents more than rearranging data bits. Therefore, questions useful in shaping the final product of autoethnography are less "what is" than "how is" and "why is." Answers are less likely to be hidden in the body of data than in your mind that processes and interacts with the data.

Quick tricks showing how to string bits of data together in a certain style and a certain structure may appear useful, especially to novice autoethnographers. However, such tricks are inadequate in producing a well-developed cultural self-analysis or a confident autoethnographer. Compelling and effective autoethnographic writing results from the careful analysis of autobiographical data, critical reflection and interpretation, and actual writing, seasoned with struggles and frustration. During the process, you will immerse yourself in the sea of data and periodically emerge from it to transcend the intimate, allowing yourself to balance between descriptive particularity and interpretive generality.

This chapter provides an array of ethnographic and autoethnographic writing samples written in different styles. You will quickly discover that no one style works for all autoethnographies. Descriptive narration prevails in some; others employ an analytical and interpretive discourse. Even in predominantly description-oriented writings a variety of styles can be embedded in the text. Whichever style you decide to adopt, you should keep in mind that the autoethnographic process, culminating in writing, ultimately seeks to interpret your life experiences from a cultural perspective.

Autoethnographic Writing as Constructive Interpretation

Autoethnographic writing engages you in a constructive interpretation process. Autoethnography is interpretive in a sense that your personal perspectives are added in all steps of research, whether in data collection where certain memories are selected, in data analysis where certain themes are probed, or in data interpretation where certain meanings are searched. It is also constructive in a way that you are transformed during the self-analytical process. As a result, autoethnographic writings interweave stories from the past with ongoing self-discovery in the present. Stories from the past are interpreted in the context of the present and the present is contextualized in the past. Freeman (2004) articulates this nature of constructive interpretation in self-writing:

> Self-interpretation is . . . an act of self-construction, or poiesis—self-articulation and self-discovery entail self-creation as well. What they also entail is the idea of development, that is, the fashioning of a new, and perhaps more adequate view of who and what one is. Far from implying that this process is somehow leading to some absolute endpoint or telos, all that is being implied is that the understanding at which one has arrived is, arguably, better—fuller, more comprehensive, more adequate—than the one that had existed previously. . . . It is a process of refiguring the past and

Kent Place 504 right next to the Jewish Community Center I attended preschool.

in turn reconfiguring the self in a way that moves beyond what had existed previously. The backward movement of narrative therefore turns out to be dialectically intertwined with the forward movement of development. (p. 77)

The "development" of self—reconfiguration, reconstruction, or transformation of self—comes through arduous self-examination. Autoethnographic writings bring this self-development process to light. Foltz and Griffin (1996) point out that the "vulnerable" exposure of self is an integral part of ethnography. Although their work does not focus on autoethnography per se, the authors understand that the involvement of self legitimizes the insertion of personal interpretation especially in postmodern ethnographic writings:

> Postmodern ethnographers reject the concept of "objective truth" and remind us that writing ethnography is cultural construction, not cultural reporting. Thus ethnographic writing is "always a construction of the self as well as of the other". . . . Since all knowledge is socially constructed, the researcher, as the instrument of data collection and interpretation, plays a central role in creating this knowledge. (p. 302)

As Foltz and Griffin point out, ethnography is not a mere reporting of culture. In the same way, autoethnography is not mere description of your life experiences. The constructive interpretation of your life is what needs to be contained in autoethnographic writing. Narrative prose is most common among a variety of writing styles and expressive formats, yet you should be aware that other experimental writings such as poetry or performance scripts have been published as autoethnography, as I discussed in Chapter 3. You need to find a good match for your interpreted story.

Typologies of Autoethnographic Writings

Earlier ethnographic writings reflected ethnographers' fervor for accurate presentation of exotic cultures. Therefore, researchers' voices were intentionally hidden behind the façade of facts and science. The portrayal of other cultures was captured in the traditional academic writing style of realism. This writing tradition has dominated anthropology and is still valued strongly. Yet the possibility of realistically representing other cultures has been seriously questioned by postmodern anthropologists such as Clifford and Marcus (1986).

Autoethnographic writing is also seen as an example of departure from conventional ethnography (Gergen & Gergen, 2002):

> In using oneself as an ethnographic exemplar, the researcher is freed from the traditional conventions of writing. One's unique voicing—complete with colloquialisms, reverberations from multiple relationships, and emotional expressiveness—is honored. In this way the reader gains a sense of the writer as a full human being. (p. 14)

Conflicts between different ethnographic orientations are reflected in Van Maanen's (1988) classification of ethnographic writings. He groups ethnographic writings into three styles: "realistic tales," "confessional tales," and "impressionist tales." *Realistic tales* refer to matter-of-fact accounts and representations that ethnographers give about people whom they have studied first hand. This is the conventionally dominant style. Realistic tales are characterized by "minute, sometimes precious, but thoroughly mundane details of everyday life among the people studied" (p. 48) and include "accounts and explanations by members of the culture of the events in their lives" (p. 49). Ethnographers who employ realistic tales tend to speak of the people they have studied with the authority of an expert. In reaction to realist ethnographers' unbashful claim of authority over other people's culture, those who practice confessional ethnography expose "how particular works [really] came into being" (p. 74) in *confessional tales*. "Personal biases, character flaws, or bad habits," which Van Maanen dubs "embarrassing," are candidly displayed to demystify the ethnographic process and to augment a "reasonably uncontaminated and pure [ethnography] despite all the bothersome problems exposed in the confession" (p. 78). *Impressionist tales* highlight "rare" and "memorable" fieldwork experiences (p. 102). If realist tales focus on the culture ("the done") and confessional tales on the researcher ("the doer"), impressionist tales present the process of studying ("the doing of fieldwork") (p. 102). In other words, impressionist tales capture impressions of people, environment, or society that ethnographers gain in the process of fieldwork.

Lightfoot's (2004) classification focuses on a different aspect of narratives: "progressive," "stability," and "regressive" development of story. These terms are used in the context of narrative analysis, not particularly with autoethnography. However, these concepts capture a variety of approaches pertaining to autoethnographic narration. *Progressive narratives* follow the pattern that "the central character undergoes a transformation that is resolved in coherence and integration" and are best illustrated by "the coming of age story" (p. 27). Life-changing autoethnographic stories are easily captured in this narrative style. Life experiences, however, are not always resolved in enlightenment or transformation. Some events or happenings are mundanely repeated without any seemingly lasting effect on self. In reality, life is more likely to be filled with these kinds of stories than a big-bang revelation. Although *stability narratives* are often presented in isolation and detachment from the broader context, you as an autoethnographer would eventually need to interpret these stability narratives in the larger context of your life. *Regressive narratives* refer to a narrative style depicting "the change over time . . . marked by increasing disintegration and incoherence." Some autoethnographic writings may contain stories of chaos, confusion, disappointment, despair, and desperation; however, the ultimate autoethnographic goal of self-discovery will force you to bring resolution to these regressive narratives.

Ellis (2004) sees autoethnographic writings as not only descriptive narratives but also creative products. Her autoethnography, *Final Negotiations* (1995), tells stories of her time spent with her partner dying of cancer. This evocative story appeals to readers' emotions. She also advocates that autoethnographers tell their stories in creative ways meaningful to them—in a form of poetry, drama, and fiction. In "performative autoethnography," a written text comes alive on stage (Denzin & Lincoln, 2000; Denzin, 2003 & 2006; Ellis, 2004; Schneider, 2005). To these scholars, this creative and aesthetic approach may present a natural departure point from traditional academic writing.

Drawing from ethnographic and autoethnographic literature from a variety of social science fields, I will discuss four different writing styles that can be applied to autoethnography: descriptive-realistic, confessional-emotive, analytical-interpretive, and imaginative-creative. Excerpts from various self-narratives illustrate these styles.

Descriptive-Realistic Writing

Description and realism may not always go hand in hand. In general, however, realistic descriptive narratives depict places, people, experiences, and events as "accurately" as possible with minimal character judgment and evaluation. Detailed descriptions add life to autoethnography. These details, even when expressed in a few simple words, draw readers to the world of the writer. Let us take a look at a simple sentence that Reverend John Pierce (cited in Phifer, 2002) wrote about his growing up in the South: "My life, like most kids' lives in the subculture of the deep South, consisted of sports and outdoor activities, fishing in the lazy bayous of Louisiana of Spanish moss and bald cypress" (p. 125). This realistic narration triggers the readers' imagination to see a little boy with a fishing pole on his shoulder searching for a sweet spot on the shores of shadowy bayous for the day's lucky catch.

In this style autoethnographic writing represents a "story," so Bochner and Ellis (1996) encourage autoethnographers to add as many details as possible to their storytelling. Their own writings are always full of details. For example, they describe their personal studies at home as follows:

> In view behind the fireplace is a second-floor loft cluttered with piles of disheveled books and papers surrounding a computer, bearing the unmistakable stamp of a professor's office. On a wooden cabinet built into the side of the fireplace sits a CD player and amplifier connected to four speakers surrounding the room. . . . Facing the fireplace is a large, round, tan couch. Behind the couch stands a mahogany bookcase in which novels, cookbooks, travel guides, photo albums . . . are spread haphazardly across the shelves. A winding stairway leads to an upstairs landing that faces the fireplace and loft across the room. Off the landing are entrances to a library and a second professor's office. Hidden from view are the piles of books, a computer, printer, fax, and copier in that office, and floor-to-ceiling bookcases in the library. The journals on the top shelves. . . . (p. 13)

The lively details of books, papers, and computer are sufficient to create the ambience of two professors' home offices. These material artifacts indicate the culture of professors wrapped about the activities of reading and writing.

For descriptive writing in qualitative research, Wolcott (1994) suggests that researchers "remove themselves from the picture, leaving the setting to communicate directly with the reader" (pp. 12–13). In autoethnography, it is not possible for you to remove yourself from the picture totally; yet it is achievable if you attempt to describe your behaviors or contexts as closely as possible to what they were, with little interjection of your opinions and evaluations. This kind of objective, realistic description can set up a context for later cultural interpretation or be interlaced with analytical and interpretive remarks.

Confessional-Emotive Writing

In confessional and emotive writing, you are free to expose confusion, problems, and dilemmas in life. Personal agonies, usually hidden from public view, are often subjects of confessional and emotive writing. Ronai's (1996) painful experience of being parented by "a mentally retarded mother" illustrates such writing:

> I resent the imperative to pretend that all is normal with my family, an imperative that is enforced by silence, secrecy, and "you don't talk about this to anyone" rhetoric. Our pretense is designed to make events flow smoothly, but it does not work. Everyone is plastic and fake around my mother, including me. Why? Because no one has told her to her face that she is retarded, . . . we don't want to upset her. I don't think we are ready to deal with her reaction to the truth. . . . I have compartmentalized a whole segment of my life into a lie. (p.110)

Like St. Augustine's *Confessions*, ground-breaking self-revealing writing from the 4th century, many confessional tales have come out of spiritual self-reflection and conversion experiences. Although not classified as autoethnography, Lamott's (2000, 2005) contemporary spiritual memoirs, *Traveling Mercies* and *Plan B*, present examples of confessional-emotive writings that contain "progressive," "stability," and "regressive" narratives in Lightfoot's terms (2004). Her stories of a happy childhood are a collection of stability narratives. When her parents got a divorce, stability and happiness in her life were dissolved into confusion, frustration, and self-destruction. These regressive narratives finally turn into progress stories as she sought a spiritual home and finally converted to the Christian faith.

Autoethnographers' vulnerable self-exposure opens a door to readers' participation in the stories. This open invitation to mutual vulnerability may appeal to readers and evoke empathy. The power of being able to speak to the hearts of readers is a natural attraction to this type of writing, according to Ellis (1996, 2004). However, confessional-emotive writings do not always enjoy favorable reviews. Rather, they are sometimes branded as emotional catharsis or "self-indulgence" because they are seen as unloading their authors' personal burdens in narration (Sparkes, 2002).

Analytical-Interpretive Writing

Analysis and interpretation are intimately intertwined but not synonymous activities in qualitative research and writing, according to Wolcott (1994). Data analysis is conducted "to identify essential features and relationships consonant with descriptors. . ." (p. 24). In analytical writing, essential features transcending particular details are highlighted and relationships among data fragments are explained. The analytical discourse, grounded in specifics, shows your ability to see interconnectedness within the case. In interpretive writing, "the researcher transcends factual data and cautious analysis and begins to probe into what is to be made of them" (p. 36). There is a danger of "reach[ing] too far beyond the case itself in speculating about its meaning or implications" (p. 37), yet you still need to look at the case in the broader context and to make sense of the relationship between your case and the context. So what is the implication of Wolcott's trinity of description, analysis, and interpretation in autoethnographic writing? His recommendation of keeping a balance among description, analysis, and interpretation in qualitative research and writing is applicable to autoethnographic writing.

An example of analytical-interpretive writing can be found in Lazarre's (1996) memoir of her experience of raising "Black" (biracial) sons as a White (Jewish) mother. Using her biracial family experience as a springboard, she analyzes implications of race in her personal life and interprets racial relations in the broader social context. She recounts her acceptance by her Black husband's family:

> I felt completely accepted by Douglas's family, and this was aided, I was later told, by my family's welcoming of them, suggesting genuineness in my capacity to love their son, *which was not automatically assumed, to say the least, of white girls dating, in love with, or marrying Blacks.* Despite the welcome, of course, I was and would always be white. (p. 44) [The italics are mine]

The italicized portion implies the social norm about interracial relationships at that time.

This descriptive writing gives a context to her later analytical-interpretive writing. As she compares her cousin's marrying a first-generation Italian American man to her own marriage to a Black man, she analyzes the societal implication of racism:

> But there are also crucial distinctions between a Jewish woman becoming part of an Italian family, an Irish man marrying into a Jewish one, even a white American of any ethnicity marrying a Nigerian or Jamaican, and a white American marrying an African American. It is a function of racism, the special white American fear and suspicion of American Blacks, that most whites simply have no idea how different African American life is from their own. Its variation, for one thing, is frequently obliterated in assumptions that all Blacks think or feel the same way about everything from politics to personal relationships. (p. 45)

The issue of racism is not yet fully developed in this brief passage. However, this writing shows the author's analytical and interpretive bent by connecting her specific case with the broader societal issue.

Mead (1972) leaves her anthropological trace of sociocultural interpretation in a description of her paternal grandmother, a retired teacher and principal, who was a tremendous influence on her intellectual and character development. She describes how her grandmother's teaching raised gender and class consciousness. These social constructs have been integrated into her other scholarly works and it is obvious that these abstract concepts are influencing the description of her grandmother in her autobiography.

> She was conscious of the developmental differences between boys and girls and considered boys to be much more vulnerable and in need of patience from their teachers than were girls of the same age. This was part of the background of my learning the meaning of gender. And just as Grandma thought boys were more vulnerable, my father thought it was easier for girls to do well in school, and so he always required me to get two and a half points higher than my brother in order to win the same financial bonus. (pp. 51–52)

Lazarre's first writing sample and the excerpt from Mead's autobiography have interpretive statements embedded in descriptive narratives, while Lazarre's second sample is written in a more interpretive style. It is possible to transition from a specific narrative style to a highly academic, analytical-interpretive discourse common in conventional scholarly writing. Nash's (2004) "personal scholarly narrative" falls in the latter style. Romo's (2004) autoethnography, included in Appendix F, balances both analysis and interpretation in this style of writing.

Imaginative-Creative Writing

The imaginative-creative writing style is the boldest departure from traditional academic writing. Imaginative energy has been channeled through a variety of genres—for example, poetry, fiction, and drama. Your creativity is the only limit to this type of experimental auto-ethnography. It opens up creative possibilities to you and imaginative participation to readers. You can express your story in less structured and inhibited formats; readers can be actively engaged in interpreting your creative expressions. This approach to writing is subject to criticism for blurring genres of fiction and nonfiction, not engaging sufficient cultural analysis and interpretation, and dismissing academic or scientific methods. Despite the criticisms, however, some social science scholars have employed it unapologetically to breathe creative energy into a portion or the entirety of their autoethnographies.

Richardson (1992) considers poetry an excellent format for auto-ethnographic writing. Having been inspired by an autobiographical poem written by her research participant, she came to believe in the power of poetry for social scientists. Tillman-Healy (1996) also adopts several autobiographical poems for her autoethnography. One of the poems, "Hear Me," expresses the emotional desperation she experienced at the age of 17 when she felt suffocated by the silence and indifference of others toward her bulimic behaviors. She asked, "Why don't you hear me?" when she was waiting for others' attention. This poem expresses Tillman-Healy's desperation clearly. Yet the poem is only a portion of her autoethnography. She later contextualizes her bulimic behaviors in connection to the U.S. culture that promotes thinness as a measure of female beauty. Her approach is a good reminder that, however creatively presented, autoethnography involves more than the presentation of problems. It explains and interprets issues emerging from your autobiographical data in connection with the social context.

Developing Your Own Style

As the variety of writing examples in this chapter illustrate, not all autoethnographers and self-narrators adopt the same style of writing. Depending on their purposes, different writers have adopted different styles and have communicated effectively with readers. Some are more conventional than others; some are more creative than others. However, this does not imply that one style is inherently superior.

Autoethnographers commonly mix different writing styles in one text. Descriptive-realist narratives may be combined with analytical-interpretive writings. Imaginative-creative style may be interlaced with confessional-emotive style within one piece of writing. In the same way, confessional-emotive style may be adopted in certain segments of an otherwise predominantly descriptive-realist text. Mixing of styles may happen in balanced portions in some cases; one style may dominate in others. Like the principle of adjusting data collection, analysis, and interpretation strategies to your research, I cannot overemphasize the importance of developing a style that fits your research purpose and your writing strengths. After all, self matters in autoethnography.

Summary

In this final chapter, I reemphasize the fact that autoethnographic writing does not merely tell stories about yourself garnished with details, but actively interprets your stories to make sense of how they are connected with others' stories. In the interpretive process, you gain new knowledge and insight about yourself and others and become transformed. In this sense, autoethnographic writing is a constructive interpretive process. Although this transformation is common, the outcome of the process is expressed in many ways. Anthropologists used different typologies to describe varied styles of ethnographic writings. Having compiled and reinvented existing typologies, I came up with four styles of autoethnographical writings: descriptive-realistic, confessional-emotive, analytical-interpretive, and imaginative-creative. I discussed each style and provided writing samples to illustrate these styles, which others such as Van Maanen (1988) had done. Although you can benefit tremendously from reading other writings, you will ultimately have to find your own style to express your interpretation of your life and its connectivity to the world.

Stigmatized in our society
- wear on our skin
- reveal to others

APPENDICES

APPENDIX A. A Bibliography of Self-Narratives: Autoethnographies, Memoirs, and Autobiographies

This bibliography, compiled with Judy Ha, contains 78 entries of book-length autoethnographies, memoirs, and autobiographies, as well as anthologies of self-narratives. Given the proliferation of self-narratives, many more books are left out than included here. Works included tend to be more contemporary and familiar to the compilers. Entries are divided into two major categories: (1) autoethnographies and (2) memoirs and autobiographies. The second category is further divided into six subcategories: memoirs and autobiographies with special focus on (1) racial, ethnic, and language issues, (2) gender and sexual orientation issues, (3) religious issues, (4) politics, social conflicts, and wars, (5) childhood memories, family relations, and growing up, and (6) disability, illness, and death.

Autoethnographies and Autoethnography-Like Self-Narratives

Self-narratives included in this section are not always identified as autoethnographies by their authors. Yet I include them in this category because they contain cultural analyses beyond self-reflection, introspection, and descriptions of people, places, or events. These are all scholarly monographs or anthologies integrating cultural analyses.

Bochner, Arthur P., & Ellis, Carolyn (Eds.). (2002). *Ethnographically speaking: Autoethnography, literature, and aesthetics*. Walnut Creek, CA: AltaMira.

Ellis, Carolyn (1995). *Final negotiations: A story of love, loss, and chronic illness*. Philadelphia: Temple University Press.

Ellis, Carolyn, & Bochner, Arthur P. (Eds.). (1995). *Composing ethnography: Alternative forms of qualitative writing*. Walnut Creek, CA: AltaMira.

Nash, Robert (2002). *Spirituality, ethics, religion, and teaching: A professor's journey*. New York: Peter Lang.

Tompkins, Jane P. (1996). *A life in school: What the teacher learned*. Reading, MA: Addison-Wesley Publishing.

Tomaselli, Keyan G. (2006). *Writing in the sand: Autoethnography among indigenous southern Africans*. Walnut Creek, CA: AltaMira.

Reed-Danahay, Deborah. E. (Ed.). (1997). *Auto/ethnography: Rewriting the self and the social*. Oxford, UK: Berg.

Memoirs and Autobiographies

Memoirs and autobiographies are predominantly narrative and descriptive. Memoirs tend to present more self-reflection and introspection on focused topics than autobiographies that chronicle the progression of events and happenings in authors' lives. Since multiple topics are interwoven in many of these writings, it is difficult to pigeonhole them into mutually exclusive categories. In an effort to help readers navigate better in the ocean of abundance, however, I here classify the writings into six subcategories mentioned earlier.

Racial, Ethnic, and Language Issues

Angelou, Maya (1969). *I know why the caged bird sings*. New York: Random House.

Antin, Mary (1912). *The promised land: The autobiography of a Russian immigrant*. New York: Houghton Mifflin.

Baldwin, James (1963). *Notes of a native son*. New York: Dial Press.

Edelman, Marian Wright (1999). *Lanterns: A memoir of mentors*. Boston: Beacon.

Haley, Alex (1996). *The autobiography of Malcolm X*. New York: Chelsea House.

Hurston, Zora Neale (1984). *Dust tracks on a road*. Urbana, IL: University of Illinois.

Kazin, Alfred (1951). *A walker in the city*. New York: Harcourt Brace.

———— (1978). *New York Jew*. New York: Alfred A. Knopf.

Laye, Camara (1954). *The dark child*. New York: Noonday.

McBride, James (1996). *The color of water: A black man's tribute to his white mother*. New York: Riverhead Books.

Momaday, N. Scott (1976). *The names: A memoir*. New York: Harper & Row.

Parks, Rosa (1992). *Rosa Parks: My story*. New York: Dial Books.

Rodriguez, Richard (1982). *Hunger of memory: The education of Richard Rodriguez*. New York: Bantam.

Walker, Rebecca (2001). *Black, White and Jewish: Autobiography of a shifting self*. New York: Riverhead Books.

Gender and Sexual Orientation Issues

Bepko, Claudia (1997). *The heart's progress: A lesbian memoir*. New York: Penguin Books.

Conway, Jill K. (Ed.). (1992). *Written by herself (volume I): Autobiographies of American women: An anthology*. New York: Vantage.

Conway, Jill K. (Ed.). (1996). *Written by herself (volume 2): Women's memoirs from Britain, Africa, Asia and the United States*. New York: Vantage.

De Beauvoir, Simone (2005). *Memoirs of a dutiful daughter*. New York: Harper Perennial.

Kidd, Sue M. (2002). *The dance of the dissident daughter*. San Francisco: HarperCollins.

Plourde, Becky (2005). *Rose of many colors*. Frederick, MD: PublishAmerica.

Religious Issues

Armstrong, Karen (2005). *Through the narrow gate: A memoir of spiritual discovery*. New York: St. Martin's Griffin.

Breyer, Chloe (2000). *The close: A young woman's first year at seminary*. New York: Basic Books.

Brooks, Ray (2000). *Blowing Zen: Finding an authentic life*. Tiburon, CA: HJ Kramer.

Carter, Jimmy (1996). *Living faith.* New York: Times Books.

Covington, Dennis (1995). *Salvation on Sand Mountain.* Reading, MA: Addison-Wesley.

Crossan, John D. (2000). *A long way from Tipperary.* San Francisco: Harper San Francisco.

Donofrio, Beverly (2000). *Looking for Mary (or, the Blessed Mother and me).* New York: Viking Compass.

Dubner, Stephen J. (1999). *Turbulent souls: A Catholic son's return to his Jewish family.* New York: Avon Books.

Goldberg, Natalie (1993). *Long quiet highway.* New York: Bantam Books.

Hathaway, Jeanine (1992). *Motherhouse.* New York: Hyperion.

Kurs, Katherine (Ed.). (1999). *Searching for your soul: Writers of many faiths share their personal stories of spiritual discovery.* New York: Schocken Books.

Lamott, Anne (1999). *Traveling mercies: Some thoughts on faith.* New York: Anchor Books.

────── (2005). *Plan B: Further thoughts on faith.* New York: Riverhead Books.

Lewis, C. S. (1956). *Surprised by joy.* New York: Harcourt Brace.

Lopez, Barry (1998). *About this life.* New York: Alfred A. Knopf.

Merton, Thomas (1948). *The seven storey mountain.* New York: Harcourt Brace.

Norris, Kathleen (1996). *Cloister walk.* New York: Riverhead Books.

────── (2001). *Dakota: A spiritual geography.* Boston: Houghton Mifflin.

Olson, Bruce (1993). *Bruchko.* Orlando, FL: Creation House.

Politics, Social Conflicts, and Wars

Ahmedi, Farah, & Ansary, Tamim (2005). *The story of my life: An Afghan girl on the other side of the sky.* New York: Simon Spotlight Entertainment.

Bonner, Elena (1986). *Alone together.* New York: Alfred A. Knopf.

Clinton, Hillary R. (2003). *Living history.* New York: Simon and Schuster.

Dau, John Bul (2007). *God grew tired of us: A memoir.* Washington, DC: National Geographic.

Gandhi, Mahatma (1957). *Autobiography: The story of my experiments with the truth.* Boston: Beacon.

Ginzburg, Eugenia S. (1967). *Journey into the whirlwind*. New York: Harcourt Brace Jovanovich.

Goodall, Jane (1999). *Reason for hope*. New York: Warner Books.

Halo, Thea (2000). *Not even my name*. New York: Picador.

Hampl, Patricia (1981). *A romantic education*. Boston: Houghton Mifflin.

Klein, Gerda W. (1995). *All but my life*. New York: Hill and Wang.

Mandelshtam, Nadezhda (1970). *Hope against hope*. New York: Atheneum.

Roosevelt, Eleanor (1984). *The autobiography of Eleanor Roosevelt*. Boston: G. K. Hall.

Childhood Memories, Family Relations, and Growing Up

Ackerley, J. R. (1975). *My father and myself*. New York: Harcourt Brace Jovanovich.

Baker, Russell (1982). *Growing up*. New York: Congdon & Weed.

Barnes, Hazel E. (1997). *The story I tell myself: A venture in existentialist autobiography*. Chicago: University of Chicago Press.

Bateson, Mary C. (1995). *Peripheral visions: Learning along the way*. New York: HarperCollins.

Bergman, Ingmar (1988). *The magic lantern*. New York: Viking.

Buechner, Frederick (1991). *Telling secrets*. San Francisco: Harper San Francisco.

Dillard, Annie (1987). *An American childhood*. New York: Harper & Row.

Doig, Ivan (1978). *This house of sky: Landscapes of a Western mind*. New York: Harcourt Brace Jovanovich.

Greene, Graham (1971). *A sort of life*. New York: Simon and Schuster.

Gosse, Edmund (1908). *Father and son*. New York: Charles Scribner's Sons.

Grumbach, Doris (1996). *Life in a day*. Boston: Beacon.

Herron, Roy B. (1999). *Things held dear: Soul stories for my sons*. Louisville, KY: Westminster John Knox.

Lott, Bret (1997). *Fathers, sons, and brothers*. New York: Harcourt Brace.

Nabokov, Vladimir (1960) *Speak, memory: A Memoir*. New York: Grosset & Dunlap.

Orwell, George (1950). *Shooting an elephant and other essays*. New York: Harcourt Brace.

Sarton, May (1968). *Plant dreaming deep*. New York: W. W. Norton.

Thoreau, Henry D. (1919). *Walden*. New York: Houghton Mifflin.

Disability, Illness, & Death

Bauby, Jean D. (1997). *The diving bell and the butterfly: A memoir of life in death.* New York: Alfred A. Knopf.

Corse, Sara (2004). *Cradled all the while: The unexpected gifts of a mother's death.* Minneapolis, MN: Augsburg Fortress Publishers.

Dubus, Andre (1998). *Meditations from a movable chair.* New York: Alfred A. Knopf.

Gunther, John (1965). *Death be not proud.* New York: Perennial Library.

Jamison, Kay R. (1996). *An unquiet mind.* New York: Vintage Books.

Kübler-Ross, Elisabeth, with Todd Gold. (1997). *The wheel of life: A memoir of living and dying.* New York: Scribner.

Peterson, Margaret K. (2003). *Sing me to heaven.* Grand Rapids, MI: Brazos.

APPENDIX B. Writing Exercises and Examples of Personal Memory Data

This appendix compiles writing exercises included in Chapter 5, Collecting Personal Memory Data, and presents selected writing samples of mine that fully or partially respond to the writing exercises.

Writing Exercise 5.1

Considering your research focus, select and chronologically list major events or experiences from your life. Include the date and brief account of each item. Select one event/experience from your timeline that led to significant cultural self-discovery. Describe its circumstances and explain why it is important in your life.

Writing Sample 5.1.1

I selected education as the main focus of my autobiographical timeline because education has always been important to my Korean family in which I grew up, my German family into which I married, and my current U.S. family which consists of two college professors (my husband and myself) and two high school students. Here is my educational history:

1959   Born into a family of educators

1966   Entered a public co-ed elementary (typical) school in the northern part of Seoul, capital of Korea

1967   Transferred to another co-ed elementary school in the southern part of Seoul

1971   Began a single-sex education (typical at the time) in the 6th grade class at the same elementary school

1972   Completed elementary school and entered an innovative, public girls' middle school that promoted self-directed learning, in Seoul

1975   Completed middle school and entered a privately owned but publicly regulated high school for college-bound girls, in Seoul

1978   Completed high school and entered an elite, private co-ed university to study education, in Seoul

1982   Completed in February undergraduate study with secondary teaching certification in ethics

1982   Began in September the M.A. program in Curriculum and Instruction with the disciplinary focus of "Anthropology and Education" in Eugene, Oregon, USA, under the tutelage of Dr. Harry Wolcott

1984   Completed the M.A. and began Ph.D. study in the same field with the same advisor

1986   Married a German doctoral student studying math at the University of Oregon, from a family of educators

1989   Completed the Ph.D. program in Curriculum and Instruction with the concentration of Anthropology and Education

1994   Started a career as a teacher educator and have remained one ever since.

Writing Sample 5.1.2

I select physical and symbolic border-crossing experiences in my life because they challenged my presuppositions and perspectives at the time they happened, have sometimes derailed me from my comfort zone, have broadened the horizon of my life, and have shaped me as a multicultural educator. Each entry identifies a border-crossing experience, then in parentheses briefly describes its effect on me.

1966   Beginning schooling (entering the world of formal and institutional education)

1971   Beginning single-sex education (entering a learning environment segregated by gender)

1976   Spiritual encounter (shifting from a parent-given faith to a self-selected faith)

1978   Entering a university in Korea (entering adulthood in the Korean context)

1982   Moving to the U.S. for graduate study (experiencing a new culture and language and a minority status in the U.S.)

1983   Learning about the sexual orientation of my academic advisor (discovering common humanity in gay persons and gaining a profound understanding of prejudice and discrimination against them)

1986   Getting married to a German (thereby adopting a third cultural and linguistic identity)

1989	Defense of my Ph.D. thesis (gaining "legal" legitimacy for practicing scholarship in the U.S.)
1989	The birth of my first child (entering a new world of motherhood)
1997	Becoming a full-time faculty (entering the world of academics and coming to terms with the power structure of higher education)
1998	Visiting Japan (overcoming age-old personal and national prejudice against Japanese)

Writing Exercise 5.2

Select a time cycle—annual, seasonal, weekly, or daily—that you want to focus on. List chronologically activities and/or events in which you participate regularly within this time cycle. Identify each item with the time framework (i.e., going to school at 7:00 am, going to church on Sunday, family visit in July/August, etc.). Briefly describe the context of such routines. Select one and describe it in detail.

Writing Sample 5.2.1

I list my annual cycle centering on a school year. As a child of educators, an educator, a spouse of an educator, and a parent of students, my life has revolved around the academic calendar and school breaks:

Aug-Sept:	Beginning of the school year
November:	Thanksgiving break
December:	Winter break & Christmas
January:	New Year's Day & the beginning of spring semester at universities
March:	Spring break at universities
April:	Children's spring break; Easter
June:	Beginning of the summer break
June-July:	Family visits or travel
August:	Church Camp for children

Summer breaks from schools are the most significant routine in my growing up as well as adulthood. I consider it typical for a traditional school culture. Having both parents as educators, I grew up with this annual downtime in summer. My husband's family, also having two teachers as parents, similarly enjoyed this yearly break. This has been a time for us to catch up with much unattended familial and professional business and take part in more leisure activities such as traveling, outdoor activities, playing music, reading for pleasure, and watching movies. Anything memorable in my childhood is associated with these summer breaks. As an adult, I associate summers with visiting relatives living afar. Symbolically, summer is for going home, the home of carefree childhood memories, parents, and siblings. Having parents still living in our homeland, the summer pleasure that our teacher parents created for us comes full circle to my children. We are paying homage to them by visiting them during summers.

Writing Sample 5.2.2

Routines in my typical workweek look like the following:

Sunday:	Church, grading, & family time
Monday:	Teaching preparation & family time
Tuesday:	Teaching & student advising
Wednesday:	Meetings, student advising, & family time
Thursday:	Teaching, meetings, & choir rehearsal
Friday:	Academic pursuits, meetings, teaching preparation, & family time
Saturday:	Children's sport activities; family time; household chores; academic pursuits

My typical week connects three dots: church, school, and home. These three elements are not neatly compartmentalized into the weekday vs. weekend paradigm. My working hours usually spill over into weekends during academic semesters. A semester is like a pressure cooker. Pressure steadily builds up for the duration of a 15-week semester until an in-between-semester break hits when pressurized steam is released all at once. Each week begins with attending church on Sunday morning. My family and I attend a Presbyterian church of over 3,500 members, which is considered "too liberal" by some Christians and "too Christian" by outsiders. Most congregants are white but the congregation makes honest but peripheral attempts to embrace people of color and reach out to communities of racial and religious diversity. Yet, congregants of color have been increasing slowly. Sometimes, I feel left to my own devices to adapt and survive in this mainline, historically "lily white" congregation. The church's social mission, music programs, and the balance between spirituality and intellectuality have pulled my family in for 17 years. I can comfortably call this my home church.

My weekdays wrap around my vocation as a college professor, filled with teaching, advising, researching, and committee meetings. Differing from research universities, the university where I teach emphasizes teaching first, service second, and research third. This priority determines routine activities that occupy my week. I spend about 40% of my working week on teaching, teaching preparation, grading, and student advising. An additional 30% is dedicated to administrative services such as meeting people, writing memos, preparing reports, and attending to other responsibilities. The remaining 30% is for other academic pursuits: reading, writing, and editing a journal.

My domestic role as a wife and mother demands considerable attention. As a typical working woman, I juggle my responsibilities to the outer world and to the domestic domain. Having spent eight years either as a full-time stay-at-home mother or part-time faculty prior to my full-time faculty position, I see both pros and cons in the world of working women. Pros and cons are unavoidable partners in my case. Professional contributions and social recognition are gratifying; however, family life and personal flexibility are often compromised in the face of work pressure.

This regimented working week is different from a typical week during breaks between semesters when family life and other academic pursuits take precedent. The noticeable difference between teaching weeks and breaks is probably typical to the life of many university professors.

Writing Sample 5.2.3

I chose to write about my typical teaching day:

The teaching profession has been my life goal since the 6th grade. Thus, a teaching day embodies my passion and identity. Two days a week, I can devote myself totally to teaching. I call them "my teaching days." I typically avoid scheduling meetings except for advising students although it is getting more difficult to do so as my administrative responsibilities have increased as Chair of Graduate Education Programs. My family understands that a teaching day is a sacrosanct day for me. Unless there is a life-threatening emergency, they do not expect me to be available from morning to midnight and

I do not plan to go home until the day is over. During the day, I typically teach undergraduate and graduate classes, prepare for teaching, meet with students, and take care of instructional office work (e.g., grading, organizing course materials, and designing on-line instruction).

Total devotion to teaching was in the air in my family when I was growing up. Having lived through the devastating Korean War, my parents considered getting college education as an absolute privilege and their teaching profession as a beacon of hope for the war-torn, poverty-stricken nation. Their parents made financial sacrifices to send my parents to school to be educated. So my parents who chose to educate other people's children guarded this life-giving privilege with stubborn commitment. I remember an occasion that illustrates my father's unwavering dedication to teaching. In the late 1970s and 1980s, student demonstrations against political dictatorship and governmental efforts to suppress the demonstrations were rampant in university campuses in Korea. In the midst of uproars, students casually skipped classes. Believing in the power of education as a catalyst of social reform and democracy, my father insisted on teaching his classes on campus even when enveloped by tear gas and noise. Even in a class where only one student showed up, he taught the full session to that one student with the same care as to an entire class. He said, "It doesn't matter how many students I have. Each one of them is just as important to educate as the whole class." His remark rings in my head as a voice of conscience when I teach and advise my students.

Writing Exercise 5.3

List five proverbs, in order of importance, that you heard repeatedly in your family, extended community, and/or society and that have had an impact on your life. Describe briefly the context in which each of them was used. Select the one most important to you and explain how it influenced your thought, belief, and behavior.

Writing Sample 5.3

Some of my childhood proverbs include:

1. Dig one well deep (used to commend or chide me to focus and excel in one area or to warn me against multi-tasking or making too many commitments for fear that I may not succeed in any)

2. Be a citizen of God's kingdom before being a citizen of Korea (used, particularly by my parents, to encourage their children to maintain their faith commitment transcending regionalism)
3. Take the golden mean (used to encourage one to take the middle ground or to discourage extreme opinions/behaviors)
4. Gather and you will live; scatter and you will die (used to encourage children to work together and to rise up together for a collectivistic or national cause)
5. Silence is golden; speech is silver (used to encourage self-reflection and self-introspection before speaking or to discourage women in particular from expressing their opinions publicly)

Writing Exercise 5.4

List five personal, familial, or social rituals, in order of importance, in which you have participated. Briefly describe the context of each ritual. Select the most important one and describe it in detail in terms of who, when, where, what, and how. Explain why it is important in your life.

Writing Sample 5.4

1. Biannual family concerts in nursing homes
2. Sunday church worship
3. Christmas eve service and dinner with friends
4. Christmas morning caroling in a local hospital
5. University graduation

One of the familial rituals I have been part of for all my life is making music together. When I was a child, we regularly sang as a family in church functions and family gatherings. Having married a person who also grew up singing and playing instruments with his family, I found it easy to carry this tradition of music making in my immediate family. With our two children, my husband and I offer family concerts of singing and playing instruments at least twice a year in local nursing homes. The ritual activities of preparation and performance follow certain steps:

1. August: setting up dates and locations of performance for the upcoming year
2. A few weeks prior to a performance date: deciding together on the program and rehearsing musical pieces

3. On a performance day: driving to the location, setting up music stands, greeting senior citizens in attendance, introducing ourselves and musical pieces, performing them, conversing with the audience, and leaving for home

Writing Exercise 5.5

List five mentors, in order of importance, who have made significant impacts on your life and briefly describe who each person is. Select one and explain how this person has influenced you.

Writing Sample 5.5

The following mentors have influenced my life in significant ways:

1. My Mother: caring mother, faithful believer, educator, professor, & trailblazer as an intelligent woman
2. My Father: education scholar and thinker
3. Rev. Young Soo Yim: Presbyterian minister in my home church in Korea, who demonstrated genuine living faith
4. Dr. Harry Wolcott: graduate program and dissertation advisor
5. Dr. Linda Stine: my neighbor and friend, copy editor, and professional colleague

My mother is one of the most important mentors in my life. She exemplifies a woman of unwavering faith, shining intellect, practical wisdom, and self-giving love, whom I try to emulate.

My mother was born in 1924 in the northwestern region of North Korea during the time of Japanese occupation. When she reminisces about her growing up in a family of both parents with six children, I can tell she had a happy childhood. Knowing that traditional and Confucian Korea placed many restrictions on women's public and domestic behaviors at that time, I'm amazed to learn how much my mother, the third child and a girl, was allowed to do. She helped her father run his orchard even as a child, was sent to a traditional school with all boys, was sent away to a different town for secondary education, and was allowed to compete in local and state running races. Now that I think of it, her family allowed her to grow up with self-confidence despite her female gender that was considered socially "inferior." I have to ask myself whether her family was unique, her family's Christian faith freed them from Confucius' social constraints, or her regional culture was not as traditional as the Seoul-centric culture with which I grew up.

Her self-confidence gave her a foundation for survival in her life marked by the oppressive Japanese imperialism, the devastating Korean War, her delayed university education as a result of the war, a challenging graduate study in the U.S., an even-more challenging return to the traditional Korea, and the lonely act as a solo female professor in her university for two decades. When growing up, I admired my mother as a professional woman who received respect from her students and colleagues, as a loving mother who modeled for me confident womanhood and efficient management of household, and a practicing Christian who demonstrated an unshakable faith and humility. She juggled immense multiple roles in her life as a professor, church officer, mother, daughter-in-law, and friend. So her balancing act was a natural sight to my childhood eyes. I occasionally felt inconvenienced by her busy involvement in many different things and absences during the day and some evenings every week. My stay-at-home nurturing grandmother filled the void, which sufficiently satisfied my basic needs. My pride in my professorial mother was greater than my sense of loss.

At the age of 82, she manages her diabetes methodically and systematically through regular exercises, controlled diet, and updating her knowledge of the disease. She reads and studies about this life-threatening disease diligently in order to overcome its possible devastating effect. This approach to her life illustrates her self-determination, self-discipline, and self-motivation.

Writing Exercise 5.6

List five artifacts, in order of importance, that represent your culture and briefly describe what each artifact represents. Select one and expound on the cultural meaning of this article to your life.

Writing Sample 5.6

1. Korean/German/English Bible: my Christian faith framed by multicultural experiences
2. Computer: my technology-oriented professional life
3. Books: my academic life

4. Sneakers: my interest in and practice of a physically active life—
    running, walking, and playing tennis
5. Cell phone: my constant need and desire to be connected with
    family and others

Writing Exercise 5.7

Create your kin-gram, including all or some key kin who have
meaningfully contributed to the shaping of your life. Your kin-gram
does not include everyone in your family tree. Describe your family on the basis of this kin-gram. Add details about individuals
included in it.

Writing Sample 5.7

(See my kin-gram in Figure 5.2.)

Here I chose to write about the overall family structure with some
details about selected individuals, focusing on the striking structural
parallelism between my Korean family and my husband's German
family:

My notion of family always contains three components: my
immediate family (husband, teen daughter, and teen son), my Korean-
side family (my mother and father, mother's siblings and their children,
and my three sisters and their families), and my German-side family
(my parents-in-law, my father-in-law's siblings and their children,
and my husband's three sisters and their families). I naturally spend
most of my time with my immediate family living in the United States,
but during summers my attention shifts to my German-side family or
Korean-side family through visits to respective countries.

As my kin-gram shows, my Korean-side family and German-side
family are remarkably parallel. My mother and my father-in-law
each have multiple siblings who keep close contact with one another.
Although my mother's siblings and their children (my cousins)
lived in different parts of Seoul, the capital of South Korea, my
first family met them regularly for holidays, church functions, and
anniversaries of her parents' deaths when I was growing up. They
still do, although no longer frequently due to their frail health and
because their grown-up children have moved away. Brothers and
sisters of my father-in-law and their children (my husband's cousins)
have scattered mostly around southern Germany but come together

to celebrate adults' "monumental" birthdays (60th, 70th, etc.) and children's and grandchildren's confirmations in the Lutheran Church (or first communions in the Catholic Church). These celebrations have been part of our upbringings, albeit in two different countries, and continue to involve us and our children whenever we can manage to participate.

Another parallel is that both my husband and I have three sisters. All but one on my husband's side is married with children. These sisters and their families are a big part of family gatherings and celebrations on each side of my family. Having grown up with three sisters who have similar age gaps among them, my husband and I, both the second born, share remarkably similar sibling dynamics.

The last parallel between my German husband's family and mine include two sets of parents who are teachers. My parents are retired as education professors, my husband's parents as math and physics teachers from a *gymnasium* (a secondary school with 5th through 13th grades). Both my husband and I grew up with the daily and seasonal routines of teachers, and now that we are both college professors, we seem to complete the mirror image of both sides.

Writing Exercise 5.8

Select a place of significance that helped you gain an understanding of yourself and your relationship to others. Draw the place, putting in as many details as possible. You may outline the place or do a realistic drawing. Identify objects and persons in the drawing when necessary. Expand this exercise to additional places. Describe the place and explain why this place is significant to you.

Writing Sample 5.8

The writing sample is given in Chapter 5.

APPENDIX C. Writing Exercises and Examples of Self-Observational and Self-Reflective Data

This appendix compiles writing exercises included in Chapter 6, Collecting Self-Observational and Self-Reflective Data, and presents selected writing samples of mine that fully or partially respond to the writing exercises.

Writing Exercise 6.1

Select a specific behavioral or cognitive topic on which you want to observe yourself. Select a manageable time frame for your self-observation and identify a recording method (narrative, structured format, or hybrid). Conduct systematic self-observation and record your observation including context information such as time, duration, location, people, occasion, and mood.

Writing Sample 6.1

(A sample is given in Table 6.1.)

Writing Exercise 6.2

Form a group of two to four people who share similar experiences with you that you want to investigate further. Meet regularly to discuss your experiences. Take notes of your exchanges. Compare and contrast your experiences with theirs. Reflect on how others' contributions to the discussion stimulate your recall of the experiences.

Writing Sample 6.2

I plan to form a focus group with two Korean female professors who work in U.S. universities and are married to non-Korean men. I plan to discuss issues regarding our professional lives as Korean immigrant females and our multicultural family lives.

Writing Exercise 6.3

List five values, in order of importance, that you consider important in your life. Give a brief definition of each in your own terms. Select the most important one and explain why it is important.

Writing Sample 6.3

1. Fairness/equality: giving the same-quality (not always same-quantity) opportunity and shares to all people
2. Faithfulness: maintaining consistent loyalty to the same principle, cause, and people even when it causes personal inconvenience and loss
3. Community-orientation: caring and being concerned about needs of others in a community
4. Honesty: truthfulness to others and self
5. Diligence/industriousness: working hard with self-driven motivation to achieve goals

Writing Exercise 6.4

Complete the culture-gram (a template is available in Appendix D). Explain three primary identities you selected and your reasons for these selections. Reflect on and write what you have learned about yourself through culture-gramming.

Writing Sample 6.4

(See my culture-gram in Figure 6.1.)

I selected three primary identities for myself: Christian, female professor, and multicultural person. My first primary identity is with Christianity, particularly Presbyterianism. I'm a fifth-generation Christian from Korea. Since Protestant Christianity was introduced by American or Canadian missionaries over a hundred years ago, it has been deeply integrated into the fabric of society. Now the religion claims close to half of the nation's population. Therefore, I can say that I am a straightforward Presbyterian by birth and conviction. I also embrace Catholic and Confucian perspectives by having married into a Catholic family and having grown up in a Korea still steeped in the traditional Confucian philosophy.

My second primary identity is a female professor. As a female who grew up in a male-dominant and traditionally gendered Korea, I fought to maintain my intellectual and professional aspiration to become a college professor against gender stereotypes and discrimination. Despite my unwavering "womanist" belief in woman's equal rights, my "traditional" value of motherhood and family is amazingly intact. I am also happy to be a mother and a wife while being a college teacher, editor, and writer.

Thirdly, I am multicultural: I'm a naturalized citizen of the United States who grew up in Korea and has lived in and frequently visited Germany as an adult. Although starting out as a monolingual in Korean, I became a Korean-English bilingual with a working knowledge of German. In addition to language and culture acquisition, my extended residence and professional existence in this country woke me up to the recognition of new identities: "Asian-American," "person of color," and an "ethnic minority." My marriage to a German man has also exposed me to the German language and culture and helped me connect with the glorious and shameful history of Germany at a personal level.

Writing Exercise 6.5

Examine your culture-gram carefully. Make a list of groups of people you are unfamiliar with, dislike, or oppose (among those who are missing from your culture-gram). Select one from your list and write who they are, why you feel the way you do, and where such feelings come from.

Writing Sample 6.5

The Japanese people were enemies in my mind for several decades because I grew up learning at home, in school, and through mass media about how they colonized Korea for 36 years and how my parents suffered under Japanese occupation. They recalled that crops were rounded up to be shipped to Japan, leaving little for Korean farmers. In an effort of cultural assimilation, the Japanese government banned the use of Korean language (the quintessential pride of Koreans) in school and public places; students were forced to change their Korean name to a Japanese one; and students and faculty were required to convert to the Shinto religion (worship of the Japanese Emperor as a divine being); toward the end of the occupation, household items made of metal were confiscated to be used for raw materials for war equipment; and some young women were rounded up to be sent away as "comfort" women (prostitutes) to Japanese soldiers.

Combined with the school's anti-Japanese history lessons and occasional media reports on public outrages toward the "unapologetic" Japanese attitude about this history, my parents' personal stories had fanned my dislike of the Japanese. I remember the contempt I felt against a group of Japanese tourists who were innocently visiting an ancient palace in Seoul.

This feeling of dislike and uneasiness lasted till my mid-thirties, when my daughter became friends with a girl from Japan who had a Japanese mother (I'll call her Tamoko, a pseudonym) and American father. During their 8 months of friendship in the United States, the girls unknowingly became ambassadors of reconciliation to me. I began to see Tamoko's genuine interest in me and the Korean culture. The relationship finally brought us together in a long-term friendship and gave me the courage to visit Japan, a country that is physically close to Korea but that is psychologically far away. During the visit, I could not totally shed the feeling of resentment against older Japanese who might have been colonizers and sympathizers of the occupation. Yet positive experiences with the Japanese surpassed my expectations, and healing began to take place. Until then I had not had courage to face head on my prejudice against all Japanese, but this backdoor approach certainly helped me to begin my transformation process. Latching onto our commonality of interracial and intercultural marriage was the first step I took. Eventually I had to acknowledge Tamoko's Japaneseness and accept her holistically. She opened the door to a new understanding of the Japanese for me.

Writing Exercise 6.6

Read a self-narrative and draw a Venn diagram to show similarities and differences between your and the author's life. Select one similarity and one difference from your diagram and describe in detail in what way you and the author are similar to and different from each other. Reflect on and analyze what you have discovered about your culture in the process.

Writing Sample 6.6

(See the Venn diagram in Figure 6.2.)

APPENDIX D. Culture-Gram: Charting Cultural Membership and Identity

Your name: _____   Date of Recording: _____

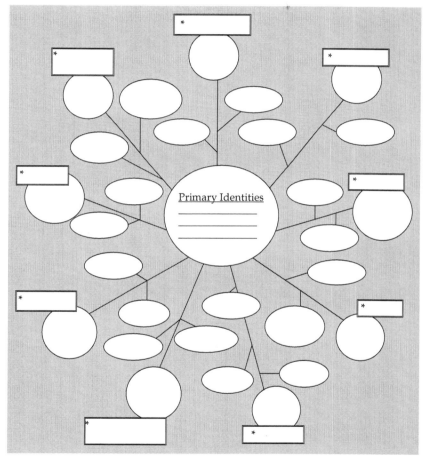

* Consider categories such as race, ethnicity, language, gender, class, religion, ability, profession, and personal interest. You may modify or expand the categories to serve your purpose.

© 2006 Chang

APPENDIX E. Writing Exercises and Examples of External Data

This appendix compiles writing exercises included in Chapter 7, Collecting External Data, and presents selected writing samples of mine that fully or partially respond to the writing exercises.

Writing Exercise 7.1

Make a list of grand-tour and mini-tour interview questions you would like to ask others about yourself, the context of your life, or other topics relevant to your study. Make a list of potential interviewees who are able to answer these questions. Select one interviewee and make a plan for an interview (name, contact information, method of interview, method of recording, and questions to ask). Conduct an interview. Take notes during the interview, and if possible, audiotape your interview. Produce the interview outcome (interview notes and/or transcripts). Make sure the interview result is clearly marked with identifiers for the purpose of recordkeeping (interviewer name, interviewee name, relationship, topic, interview method, time, and location).

Writing Sample 7.1

My interview questions are as follows:

1. Grand-tour Question: Please describe what you remember of me at our first meetings in Eugene, OR (Judy W., Ray W., Harry W., & Letty L.)
   a. Mini-tour: How was my English?
   b. Mini-tour: What was your first impression of me?
   c. Mini-tour: How did I present my Korean identity?
2. G: How have I changed since I left Korea? (Miok & Hee Young)
   a. M: How does my Korean language sound?
   b. M: Do you see any change in my view of Korea?
   c. M: How has our relationship been changed?
3. G: Please tell me what you have noticed about my adaptation to German life. (Mutti [sister-in-law] & Gerhard)

a. M: Please describe our first meeting. How did I communicate in German?
b. M: What do you think I have learned most about the German life?

Writing Exercise 7.2

Make a list of textual artifacts that you are interested in collecting. For each item identify artifact type, the time and context of its production, access (possible location, contact person, etc.), and data collection date. Select one item and locate the artifact. Describe the artifact and explain what it is for and why it is important to your life.

Writing Sample 7.2

1. My diary from my high school days (I have it in my possession)
2. Letters I sent to my parents from Eugene, OR between 1982 and 1986 (I have them)
3. Report cards from elementary through high school (I have them)
4. My journals between 1982 and the present (I have them)
5. My travel logs to Ireland, England, Russia, Brazil, and Turkey (I have them)
6. My Christmas letters from 2001 through 2005 (I have them)

Writing Exercise 7.3

Make a list of categories of nontextual artifacts that you plan to collect for your study. Make the categories broad enough, but not so broad as to be unmanageable. For example, you'll want to list a category as "photos from high school" instead of "photos." Collect artifacts that fit the category. Sort your artifacts into subcategories. Describe briefly the artifacts in one subcategory (type, time and location of its production, others represented by the artifacts, etc.) and write your reflection on the significance of these objects in your life.

Writing Sample 7.3

I will collect nontextual artifacts from the following categories:

1. photo albums
2. household objects that I use regularly that represent Korean, German, & U.S. culture
3. artifacts that represent my professorial vocation
4. my children's stuff (athletic, musical, and academic items)
5. a list of gifts that I have received or given to relatives and friends within the most recent year

Writing Exercise 7.4

On the research topic you selected, make a list of subtopics of which you plan to obtain contextual information. Draft a literature review plan including your main research topic and subtopics. Select one subtopic and conduct a preliminary literature search. If necessary, modify your literature review plan along the way. Take notes during the literature review.

Writing Sample 7.4

(See my literature review map in Figure 7.1.)

APPENDIX F. Autoethnography Example by Jaime J. Romo

Experience and Context in the Making of a Chicano Activist
From THE HIGH SCHOOL JOURNAL, Volume 87 Issue 4, pp. 95–111.
Copyright © 2004 by the University of North Carolina Press. Used by permission of the publisher. www.uncpress.unc.edu

This paper examines the experiences and context in the making of a Chicano activist. Utilizing autoethnographic methodology, I discuss my own identity development, as it was mediated by issues of social capital and mentoring, two significant elements related to Chicano educational activism. I discuss dimensions of race, class, self-esteem, and professional development as they relate to transformative educators and activism.[1]

Key Words: mentoring; transformation process; autoethnography; identity development

Overview

Upon examining the literature on teachers and change, two alarming facts emerge. First, the overwhelming majority of teachers continue to be White or European American and tend to teach in the way that they learn (Romo, Bradfield, & Serrano, 2004). Secondly, we have classrooms with diminishing numbers of students who are European American. A crisis is looming: many teachers misunderstand, marginalize and mis-serve the growing minority-majority population by teaching and interacting with students as if students shared in the teachers' backgrounds. Concurrently, a virtual academic industry has developed related to European American teachers and students under-standing their whiteness as it relates to teaching and learning (Delpit, 1995; Howard, 1999; Kohl, 1994; McIntosh, 1989; Scheurich, 1993; Scheurich & Young, 1997; Sleeter & McLaren, 1995). Despite a growing body of knowledge about teachers who practice educational social justice, much more needs to be understood about the lives of Chicano/Latino students and teachers (Fredrickson, 1995; Moll et al., 1993; Romo, Bradfield, & Serrano, 2004). Therefore, it is necessary to consider alternative educational social justice practitioners' voices in order to break the following patterns.

The dropout rates across the nation for Latinos, African Americans, and American Indians are particularly high (Kitchen, Velasquez & Myers, 2000) when compared to European American students. In the U.S., dropout rates for Latinos and American Indians hover between 40 and 50%, almost double that for African Americans and triple that for whites. In other words, out of one hundred White students that enter kindergarten, ninety-three earn a high school diploma, sixty-five attend at least one year of college, and thirty-four complete a B.A. degree. Of one hundred Black students that enter kindergarten, eighty-seven earn a high school diploma, fifty-one attend at least one year of college, and seventeen complete a B.A. degree. However, out of one hundred Latino students that enter kindergarten, sixty-three earn a high school diploma, thirty-two attend at least one year of college, and eleven complete a B.A. degree. Among Native Peoples, only fifty-eight percent complete high school and seven percent attend at least one year of college (Haycock, 1997; The Education Trust, 1998).

We know that the quality of teaching is the most important determinant of student success (Darling-Hammond, 1998; Elmore & Burney, 1997) that leads to student success or its antithesis, sharecropper education (Moses, 2001). However, students of color report that white, ethnically encapsulated teachers: did not know them nor did they care to; were biased against students' cultures; and were insensitive to issues they faced at home (Kitchen, Velasquez & Myers, 2000). Schools, in truth, often felt like prisons by students who faced cultural discontinuities and personal and institutional racism on a daily basis (e.g., Chávez Chávez, 1995, 1997; Delpit, 1995; Kitchen, Velasquez & Myers, 2000).

By looking at K-12 educational system as a whole, it is possible to conclude that, as a society, we are all complicit in the miserable learning conditions and outcomes related to Latino students (Darder, Torres, & Gutierrez, 1997; Howard, 1999; Kozol, 1994). For example, how is it that while the proportion of Latinos in the United States increases, the number of Latinos who complete graduate degrees, particularly doctorates decreases (Gonzalez et al., 1998)? I believe that by understanding Chicano educational activist educators, people who promote individual, interpersonal and institutional transformation towards equity and inclusion in a multicultural society, we can better serve the growing minority-majority student population. Therefore, this study hopes to provide insights into the questions: What factors influence the development of Chicano educational activists? How does Chicano activism in higher education relate to K-12 educational practices for all students?

The following autoethnographic study allows for a rich vein of anecdotal information about schools, identity development, mentoring and activism that traditional quantitative or ethnographic methodologies can miss (Bochner, 1997; Ellis & Bochner, 2000). In this study, I examine my experiences, as a representative of a nationally small group of Chicano professors/activists, to extend understandings of the dynamics related to the makings of a Chicano advocate (Reed-Danahay, 1997). The study offers readers a glimpse into the "totality" of the experiences involved in the making of a Chicano educational activist by utilizing racial identity development and social capital theory as well as current research on transformative teaching (Bourdieu, 1977; Romo, Bradfield, & Serrano, 2004; Romo & Roseman, 2004; Tatum, 1998).

Methodology

I chose an auto-ethnographic methodology as an approach to examine my own development as a Chicano activist because, as Tierney states, "auto-ethnography confronts dominant forms of representation and power in an attempt to reclaim, through self-reflective response, representational spaces that have marginalized those of us at the borders" (1998, p. 66). Autoethnography is a genre of writing and research that connects the personal to the cultural, placing the self within a social context (Reed-Danahay, 1997). These texts are usually written in the first person and feature dialogue, emotion, and self-consciousness as relational and institutional stories affected by history, social structure, and culture (Ellis & Bochner, 2000).

The context of autoethnography as a research method in this study is that those with power are frequently least aware of or least willing to acknowledge its existence as well as their role in maintaining inequitable social and cultural capital that leads to student marginalization (Delpit, 1995; Stanton-Salazar, 1997, 2001). In fact, Paulo Freire (1985) would say that, because of privilege, dominant culture members actually resist change toward equity. Therefore, it is highly appropriate that an autoethnographic approach is utilized to examine Chicano experiences in education, through a Chicano researcher's presentation of findings (Charmaz & Mitchell, 1997; Holt, 2003).

I originally generated this data approximately eighteen months ago for my undergraduate and graduate teacher education students. This was a way to help them know more about their instructor's emphasis on their becoming multi-culturally competent advocates for all children. It was an autobiographical written narrative depicting my experiences as a student and educator that was based upon years of reflections on identity, voice, recovery and purpose. The essay also modeled part of a self-reflexive final project that dealt with a final educational philosophy project. I tried to produce an account of identity development and significant experiences related to my trajectory as an educational activist, particularly for marginalized students.

As a result of continuous reading and rereading, long after writing the initial narrative, I identified units and then categories from the data. Four key categories emerged from the data: The bittersweet context of school; Chicano identity development; Mentoring; and stages of growth as an activist.

Findings

This examination began with the following questions: What factors influence the development of Chicano educational activists? How does Chicano activism in higher education relate to K-12 educational practices for all students? The data offered several insights to these questions, as well as some links for teacher educators and K-12 educators to consider in their work.

The Bittersweet Context of School: Hope and Wounding

Across the nation, a growing number of children are born into poverty. They enter kindergarten with hopes and dreams of opportunity, progress, and dreams fulfilled. Unfortunately, by the time most leave school, many of their hopes have withered—dried up like raisins in the sun. The social class of poor students consists of "black, Hispanic, and Asian class fractions, together with the white aged, the unemployed and underemployed, large section of women, the handicapped, and other marginalized economic groups" (McLaren, 1994, p. 180). In the United States, this underclass continues to increase as access to the privileges held by the middle and upper class diminish. And, despite the "myth of meritocracy" that maintains that a solid work ethic is all one needs to pull her/himself up "by her/his bootstraps," the U.S. middle class is diminishing, the upper class remains relatively static and the underclass is growing. About 25% of U.S. children live in poverty and that percentage continues to increase (Romo, Bradfield, & Serrano, 2004).

Schools in rural or urban poverty-stricken neighborhoods have a particularly significant opportunity to make or break underclass children. If such schools are not proactive in mitigating the negative impacts poverty can have on children who grow up poor, they can negatively impact children's lives (e.g., Books, 1994; McDermott & Rothenberg, 1999, 2000; Payne, 1998). For example, schools with large populations of poor children often have policies and practices that reinforce compliance, obedience and passive intake of knowledge (Anyon, 1980a, 1980b; Anyon & Wilson, 1997). These become the background for the overall context of school as a set of bittersweet experiences for many Chicanos, emerging educational activists, and the following two reflections.

It was a sunny, September Friday in 1965. My first grade class at Divine Savior Elementary School in Cypress Park, in northeast Los Angeles, was gearing up for our weekly spelling competition. Our orderly room with the pretty bulletin boards, chairs in precise rows, and friendly mice and frogs in their cages on the bookshelf against the wall had become a second home to me. My first home wasn't like the neat, controlled environment, where I got consistent feedback, attention, praise, and sometimes hot dog, cupcake and chocolate milk on a Friday.

Within a few months, I had become the champion speller in my class. The Friday spelling contest was my stage, and I nervously sat, fully immersed in spelling colors and numbers, awaiting my turn to reestablish my spelling championship status, whatever it cost. Jeannie Prudell was a good speller and we were in a championship spell-off in my classroom. Jeannie Prudell was the first White girl I had ever met. On the first day of school, we were lined up: Ortega, Prudell, and Romo. The heavy, blonde, blue-eyed White girl, turned around and for no apparent reason declared, "I can spell stop: S-T-O-P. I can spell yellow: Y-E-L-L-O-W." My mother, unlike lots of my classmates' moms, had already taught me to read well, but still I thought that Jeannie Prudell must have been a genius because she knew so much that she couldn't hold it in.

Sister called me to the board to spell the next word, but I also had to go to the bathroom. The contest won out and I marched to the board to spell orange: O-R-N-G-E, as I quietly peed on myself, leaving a small puddle for the next student to discover and declare, "Ooh, sister, somebody peed!" It wasn't such a big deal in itself, but for me, who wanted so early to be so perfect, it was a symbolic act: I was a spelling, peeing paradox, sitting in a pool of shame. At age six, the primacy of academic performance meant more to me than meeting my own basic physical needs. I loved school and achievement more than myself, so I wouldn't give up my spot in the contest, my moment to shine, or admit that I had a need. What a foreshadowing of my years of teaching, wherein I held my pee like a pro, like all good teachers do, for the sake of the craft.

The first quote illustrates the socio-cultural gaps that often exist between classrooms and students' home environments. Despite early academic accomplishment, I exhibited a kind of adulation that many students of color pay to dominant culture members. The second quote highlights the compliance that I had internalized, partly related to Mexican culture 'respeto,' and partly related to the explicit authority that religion and religious figures made explicit in school.

A context of school as bittersweet frames the overall experiences of Chicanos and other students of color in schools. For me, this continues to be an accurate description of my experiences as a teacher, a K-12 administrator and university professor. However, I now have the benefit of a more developed and integrated identity, understanding of educational and societal dynamics, and mentoring that I discuss in the following sections.

Identity Development

Frameworks of racial/ethnic identity development generally work from a lower to higher level, whether they relate to dominant culture members (Hardiman, 1982; Helms, 1990; Howard, 1999), ethnic people of color (Atkinson, Morten, & Sue, 1989; Cross, 1991; Kim, 1981; Solis, 1981) or biracial or bicultural individuals (Poston, 1990; Stonequist, 1961[1937]). Similar to other developmental models, growth varies based on context and experiences. In the case of racial/ethnic identity development, sociopolitical and contextual factors create conditions which could prevent internalizing a normalized identity and, at times, arrest normal progression. In the following examples, we see how racial identity development intersects with class and psychological or self-esteem conflicts, before yielding an integrative stage of identity.

Identity development: racial dimensions Prior to meeting Jeannie, I was unsure about what White people were like. My prior experience was only through TV and TV made me very conscious of what the 'good life' meant, and how my family didn't have it or look like those who did. School was my way of entering into a slice of this good life that, while not my own, was where I was liked and accepted by some White teachers and some White kids.

Most of the kids were Latinos, first or second-generation Mexicanos, but the few White kids stood out to me as parts of the world I saw on TV. Rick Jones, a blonde, crew cut sporting White boy gave me another pleasant experience with White people. A week before my fateful Friday spell-off, some classmates were spinning tops at recess. We'd throw our tops and then pick them up and let them continue spinning in our hands. Danny Olivas crouched down to pick up his top and right as the metal top tip was at the point of contact of the web between his two fingers, I threw my top. I didn't mean to throw it near him, but it happened to hit his top, which pinched his hand. He jumped up and charged me. Out of nowhere, Rick Jones jumped in between us, pushed Danny and said, "Hey, leave my friend alone." I watched in surprise that this White boy would call me his friend and stand up for me. While Rick may not have any thought of race at that point, I did. It was a subtle consciousness that came up every once in a while, mostly when I saw TV.

At the same time, every time a school person said my name, I got a consistent message that I was unusual or foreign. In its apparent innocence, it was a pattern of not being seen as I am. My mom named my five siblings and me so that we'd keep our names in English and Spanish: Leticia, Conrad (named after our father, Conrado), Jaime, Marina, Rene and Teresa. I think she must have known how important was the idea of keeping our names, which represented our identities and our connectedness to our past. She assimilated in lots of ways, yet she maintained a connection to her language, relatives in Mexico, and community; still, her inclusion as Vangie or Lina seemed like a mainstream way to see her as White, as "Latina-lite." Her name was Maria Evangelina.

/Jay-me/ is what I get when most people see my name spelled J-a-i-m-e. I guess that there's a Jamie and Jaime spelling that some people claim as /Jay-me/. As a child or as an adult, when a non-Latino has wanted to be friendly, he's said, "Hi-me, that's my name—Jim." Even as a child, I knew that my name is Jaime, not hi-me and not Jim. Santiago is James, Santiaguito might be Jim. Being re-named by others represents years of absorbing people's misinterpretations or impositions. For years, I smiled, I was nice and I didn't want to offend. I put up with and excused others, even though it felt bad, because I believed that it was flattering to be given the attention. But my name represents the core of who I am. And who I am represents something that others needed to change in order to relate to me.

The previous quotes reflect the assimilationist context that people of color often experience in schools and in society. Valenzuela (1999) argues that schools, in fact, have a subtractive nature by minimizing students' language and culture. Therefore, a sign of post-assimilation racial identity development for people of color is to reclaim names or other ethnic markers in order to both reject the assimilation and claim their own identity (Atkinson, Morten, & Sue, 1989; Cross, 1991; Kim, 1981; Solis, 1981). The expression for "What's your name?" in Spanish is "Como te llamas?" ("What do you call yourself?"). What we call ourselves says a lot about how connected we are to our roots, ethnicity, and language of origin. It often takes a conscious effort to keep those connections through names in an assimilationist society. When my first son was born, my father and sister chided me for not naming Jesus something more 'mainstream,' like Michael Francis. This speaks to the discomfort so many Latinos feel about being ethnic in a society that despises Latinos, as well as the desire and fantasy that so many carry to be mainstream.

Identity Development: Class Dimensions Public schools generally have at least three tracks of classes and over-place poor students (of color) in academic tracks beneath their actual ability level (e.g., tracking) due to preconceived notions of performance. Consequently, social class becomes a powerful filter that practically defines who succeeds and who does not. Students' self-esteem is often permanently affected as perceptions of their academic abilities and future possibilities dry up over time (Romo, Bradfield, & Serrano, 2004). Many Chicanos experience the bitterness of not fitting in to school environments. Since I experienced some academic and athletic success in school, I persisted. However, many others turn inward (Tatum, 1998) and subsequently find themselves disconnected from the educational gatekeepers and resources that can help Chicanos resist assimilation or identity loss and find school success (Stanton-Salazar, 1997, 2001). In the following section, I examine how attending a private, elementary school, college prep high school, and university influenced my identity development.

For me, school was where I was safe, where I felt valued, included, liked, and successful. But no place is completely safe and sometimes the violence from the neighborhood carried over to the church property and a normally safe parish fiesta exploded. The crowded schoolyard was lined with food and game booths and families swarmed the property; "I'm your Puppet" blared for the twentieth time that day from the jukebox in the corner near the snow cone booth. A few feet away from me, someone from another neighborhood must have bumped someone from a Cypress Park clique and within seconds, a group surrounded the unlucky intruder and kicked and beat him to the ground. Nonetheless, I generally felt safe at school and it was there that I got picked to go on the Art Linkletter Show in 1966. Art was a gentle, friendly man who knew Sister Monroe, the principal of my grammar school. He, no doubt, asked her to supply gullible, obedient children who would sincerely answer questions, even if we had no idea what the questions or answers meant. All I knew was that I felt special because I got picked. My three classmates and I got to the studios and played in the waiting room for the taping to begin. The waiting room was carpeted and had cool toys that I didn't have, like "A Barrel of Monkeys." While I played, some television people primed us with questions in a friendly, conversational way. "What do you like about school?" I told them about some cool frogs we had in the classroom. "What do you want to be when you grow up?" I didn't know. I don't think anyone had asked me that before first grade. So when I got under the hot studio lights and Art Linkletter asked me what I wanted to be when I grew up, all I could think of was how cool it was to have those frogs in the classroom and how I could make that happen for other kids. The stagehands may have mentioned veterinarian back stage, but all that came out of my mouth was, "I want to be a tadpole keeper." Everyone laughed. Backstage, another question was, "If you were president of the United States, what would you do?" I didn't know what presidents did, but the stagehands asked, "Would you run for second term? . . . Would you run for third term?" Sure. I figured that if they asked, there must be such a thing, and that if two is good, three is better. I was the supposed smart kid in the class and I had fallen for the backstage set up. So when Art asked, "If you were president of the United States, what would you do?" I was ready. "I'd run for third term." Everyone in the audience laughed again, and I had no idea what I had said. Our pay for being goobers on national television was a limousine ride to the famous Beverly Hills restaurant, The Brown Derby, to feast on a huge ice cream sundae or banana split, either of which were heaven on earth for me.

School was my oasis and sometimes my mirage. When I was in the eighth grade, I still wet the bed and was still terrorized by the violence in my home. When I heard about a private high school that had boarders, I knew that I had to get a scholarship to attend and get away from my house and the insanity I lived in. I'd often go to bed dreaming of living in the boarding house, without cockroaches, crashing furniture or piercing screams in the middle of the night that would transform me into Mighty Mouse, my favorite after school cartoon character, to save someone or into the invisible man so I could hide and be safe. I wanted out of my house and school was going to be my boarding ticket. I knew (or maybe was so desperate and unaware of any other alternatives) that doing well in school would help me—somehow, in some way, someday. With good grades, I thought, I could be a lawyer and defend kids, like the kids I grew up with who didn't seem special to anyone and who got into trouble. That dream propelled me through many all-nighters at a young age wherein I'd finish every assignment, no matter how tired I was. In high school, I obeyed school authorities and rules, I never challenged or spoke back to teachers, and I was a decent high school soccer player. High school was a place where I could channel my anger in constructive, socially acceptable ways. Besides getting good grades, I got a mysterious pleasure at beating rich White boys in the classroom. That was my consolation when, every day, my efforts to fit in, to look like, sound like, and act like my wealthier White peers dissolved like a mirage when I got home.

At school, I'd overhear their stories about their dates over the weekend, driving their convertible to the racetrack or to some expensive concert and I'd feel jealous. At the same time, they gave me my model for what dates are supposed to be like. As a senior, I met a young woman from a girls' school at a dance and later, we went out on my first date. I wanted to go out and live like my schoolmates. I borrowed a car from my molester priest, and I wore the leisure suit and polyester shirt he had bought for me when he took me to Hawaii, like I was a prince for a day. I really liked the young woman, but I never called her again. I felt terrible that we lived in polar opposite socio-economic worlds and that I couldn't afford to date her. Besides, I only had one leisure suit. Again, my illusion of school as the great equalizer that would override my miserable home life left me. So when the mirage faded, it was a bonus that I outperformed lots of rich, White boys in the classroom and on the field.

When it came time to apply to colleges, I filled out my own financial aid forms. Mom left the financial matters to my father and he left them to me. While I could figure out paperwork, I was under-prepared for managing my life in such a fast paced, high-powered environment as Stanford offered. As successful as I was in a college preparatory high school, my leap into Stanford life was disorienting and fostered nagging questions that lead to insecurity. This insecurity was a kind of not being at ease (dis-ease) with the core of being who I was. As a result, I floundered through my undergraduate education.

Of the many class issues to develop, I will highlight three that emerge from the data: cultural capital, violence and symbolic violence, and a migratory identity development. Cultural capital refers to what middle and upper class families pass on to their children, which substitutes for or supplements economic capital as a way of maintaining class status and privilege (Bourdieu, 1977). Gonzalez et al. (2003) discusses how low-income and underrepresented students do not sufficiently possess the knowledge of what college is, the diversity of institutions, the admissions process, graduation rates of different types of institutions, or utility of various degrees. This theme of limited cultural capital expected in mainstream institutions and the experience of being under prepared for social or academic rites of passage relates to my own memories.

While some parents can pass on middle-class cultural capital, others pass it on with violence or the symbolic violence of exclusion, marginalization and classism (Nieto, 2000). The U.S. Census Bureau notes that approximately 37% of children in the United States today live in poverty. Popular wisdom suggests that many more families live one check away from homelessness, like I did. Children enter kindergarten with hopes and dreams of opportunity, progress, and dreams fulfilled. Unfortunately, by the time most leave school, many of poor children's hopes have withered—dried up like raisins in the sun. In the quotes, it is clear that I persevered through a violent home, a violent neighborhood and the symbolic violence of not having enough and not feeling as if I were enough in middle and upper class academic environments.

The last theme from these class memories is that of a migratory identity. Given the poverty of local public schools, my parents sacrificed and sent me and my siblings to private schools. For me and many students to participate in prestigious and rigorous educational programs, we have to leave the neighborhood and often separate from our friends and support group. Later in this discussion, I raise the image of being a professional migrant worker as an empowering identity descriptor. However, in these formative years, I felt more isolated and pressured to disconnect from my roots, or connect in an intellectual way, knowing that I represented others who sacrificed for me to have more opportunities than they had.

Identity Development: Self Esteem Conflicts Positioning theory notes that as we take up a position assigned to us by others, we begin to see the world from the vantage point of that position. In the following memories, I took up the 'good student' role, even when it did not seem to produce the benefits of academic success or even led me to the shameful contrasts of hopes and experience.

"Ooh, sister, somebody peed!" . . . I was pretty embarrassed, but the teacher and my mom were very gentle with me. I'm sure that the teacher had seen this many times in her career, so it wasn't a big deal for her. My mom, on the other hand, probably thought that this was a continuation of my bed wetting at home most nights. She knew that I was so damned scared of my dad's drinking and violence that I slept in a stinky bed and kept a stinky secret with her for many years. But my mom didn't know about my other grammar school secrets that I carried: the fact that I was molested by the parish priest and his friend; the fact that I was ashamed of my poverty and home for so many years; the fact that at some point I transferred the shame of what wasn't perfect about what happened to me to who I was.

This is an example of what qualitative research can uncover that quantitative research cannot (Bochner, 1997; Ellis & Bochner, 2000). The pain and shame I felt as a child from my home life was compounded by the devastation of molestation by a religious authority figure. For various reasons, many Chicanos feel ambivalent about school and authority figures. Some feel the symbolic violence of rejection or manipulation by teachers or other authority figures (Nieto, 2000). The juxtaposition of these home and school experiences illustrates how Chicanos and other students of color contend with or resist a lifetime of symbolic violence and/or ambivalence about school.

These memories also elicit a tone of desperation and failure. As a student and professional, the hard work and sacrifice I invested in school seemed to draw the proverbial check marked 'insufficient funds' when it came time to enjoy the benefits of academic achievement. While these memories may seem devastating, they are also the foundation of activism that I will discuss in later sections of this article.

Identity Development: Integration Examinations into the lives of educational activists (Romo, Bradfield, & Serrano, 2004; Romo & Roseman, 2004) have uncovered that activists: have questioned their own mindsets, have experienced cultural dissonance, have experienced the pain caused by both the actions of misinformed others, and have begun to face their own demons grounded in their privilege and/or biases. All, however, continue to struggle in the everyday as advocates for their students. The following narratives represent a kind of personal and professional integration that comes through practice.

I identify with brown men who wait for work on supermarket corners—men who will break their backs for a day's wage and say thank you. It takes guts to stand on street corners waiting for someone to come and offer you a job, meanwhile hoping that the INS won't pick you up to send you away from here, away from where there's work that can take care of your family. It takes courage and tenacity to sleep in hills or wherever is affordable and then to clean up to be presentable to ask for work out in public. It takes faith and endurance and resistance and persistence to show up every day and sacrifice food, comfort, and family, to live and work alone among strangers.

Brown men and women wait for work in strawberry fields and in educational fields—men and women who will break their backs for a day's wage and say thank you. It takes deep faith that somehow God will take care of us and our loved ones as we do the best we can do, without contacts, without understanding the hidden culture of the system, and without support. It takes great heart to stand amid disdain and hatred and not lash back when people blame us for taking their jobs away, for not being qualified to be where we are, for making them feel uncomfortable and be dependent on someone else's prerogative to select.

I'm a migrant worker with more education, more possessions, more visions of changing the systems that perpetuate dark people waiting on corners for work. Because of my journey of poverty and temporary assignments, I am an advocate for social justice through teacher education. Because I know what it is like to be marginalized, isolated, and rejected [as a professional], I organize Latino faculty and staff to help themselves and empower others to find a place at the educational table and institutionalize equity and diversity.

Part of my empathy for kids in elementary or middle school in particular comes from the secret hell I lived that taught me how much energy it takes to keep secrets. I empathize with kids who put on a happy face when angry or terrified because they don't know how to handle the monsters that are real (Edelman, 1992).

Scholars report that Latinos/as and American Indians remain the most underrepresented major ethnic groups at institutions of higher learning—especially at selective, four-year liberal-arts colleges and research universities—as students, tenured professors, and academic administrators. In addition, key decision makers in the selection process for presidents and provosts expected higher standards of qualifications and experience for Latino men and women than for members of other ethnic and racial groups (Haro, 1995). It is with my experiences in mind that I work to redeem my own life experiences and transform the conditions that perpetuate experiences of inequity, marginalization and violence for others.

My personal and professional integration process has paralleled my ethnic/racial identity development process. Overall, I have come from rejecting my home experience and culture in order to assimilate and be accepted into the mainstream, to embracing my heritage with a vengeance (rejecting anything that represented dominant culture), to negotiating the knowledge, dispositions, and skills from both worlds.

When I recall the image of migrant worker, therefore, it is with a personal identification with migrant Latino families, even though I now hold a middle class professional cultural capital. It is with this perspective that I can better understand my mentoring experiences as well as my work as an activist, which I discuss in the following sections.

Mentoring

In a study of 14 Latino educational administrators, one theme was clear: the need for mentors and mentoring of Chicano students to develop future educational activists in both teaching and administration (Romo, 1998). My activism, particularly as a Chicano, has been shaped through both negative and positive mentoring experiences, although the predominant experience of professional mentoring has been a lack of mentoring. The following sections illustrate how this mentoring looked, sounded, and felt in my educational experiences.

Negative Mentors

The experiences of . . . longing began my search for a mentor, a successful authority who could validate me with my experience and my perspective, as well as my [Spanish] name. I can't overstate how significant the lack of mentoring I experienced was in my formative years. Until I had my own sense of being an author and authority of my own experience, I constantly questioned myself: "Am I somehow bringing something that's true, or real, or that makes sense to others?" And the making sense meant looking for someone to validate me. The making sense meant looking for someone who was successful and 'authoritative,' yet enough like me that I could trust her/his judgment and benefit from her/his authoritative voice when it spoke to my merit, my place, my authenticity.

As an undergrad in a predominantly white institution, I never knew my assigned advisor and after trying a series of majors, I found a Latino professor in the history department who agreed to be my advisor. At the beginning of my last quarter, I met with him. "Any suggestions on what I should do next?" I asked, unsure of myself and aware that I had pieced together a history degree. "Well, I wouldn't suggest that you be a historian." I'm sure I was reaching for nurturing or empathy from a fellow Latino, who represented an idealized intellectual father figure to me. My blind faith and dreams propelled me for years in my search for a mentor, someone who had been where I wanted to go, someone who even looked like me. I was profoundly embarrassed, more so than in my peeing, spelling debacle. More than in front of a national television audience who laughed at me because I didn't understand the questions. I filed away my numb self-esteem, got drunk and determined that I would redeem myself someday. I wasn't surprised, when I received my diploma from Stanford, that the reader called out another version of my name, "Jaime Who-deh (Jude) Romo."

Positive Mentors

In high school, two teachers pushed me to achieve and I responded to them because I sensed that they valued me and my name. Perhaps it helped that they called everyone by last name, so for the first time, teachers pronounced my name correctly. Fr. Eugene Colosimo was a feisty Sicilian Jesuit who refused to accept minimal effort or results from me in his Algebra and Trigonometry courses. Mr. Pat Rowell was a gentle White English teacher who told the class about his Latina wife's experiences of poverty in her formative years. By acknowledging that he appreciated struggle, I worked especially hard in his class. Despite their and others' support, I was without a mentor.

I entered Stanford in the fall of 1977 with two Chicano high school friends. They each had a plan and did well. [One] was a wealthy Chicano, whose father was a General Practitioner and who owned a large ranch in Mexico. He knew what it took to get into medical school from day one. He knew the language, culture, system and schedule. He worked hard and went from Stanford to USC medical school. [The second] was interested in being a lawyer and he also had a plan and worked hard. During our senior year, [my second friend] and I met on campus and he announced that he had just gotten his LSAT scores. "Great. How'd you do?" I asked. "Pretty good." He replied before adding, "For a Mexican." We both laughed at our insecurity and struggle to succeed. He went on to UCLA law school.

Finally, after six years as a teacher and twenty-three years as a student, I found a Chicano mentor. It was during my final assistant principal interview with Superintendent of Sweetwater Union High School District, Julian Marta. He surprised me when he asked, "What are you going to say to the teacher who says, 'The reason you got this job is because you are Latino and the superintendent is Latino'?" We engaged in a role-play discussing my qualifications. He then said to me, "Are you willing to work longer hours than everybody else, work harder and do a better job than anyone else? If you are, then the job is yours." I was surprised, not by his questions, but by his openness regarding his Latino experience in the context of White privilege. He knew that for people of color to be respected and effective, we have to do more than anyone. He was an honest mentor and I appreciated his validation of my professional worth. He was a Stanford graduate, too. He also knew that I knew that school is very different for lots of poor kids, especially students of color. His presence and example empowered me to advocate for kids who succumb to the intolerance, the racism, the hatred, misunderstandings, physical dangers in schools and society, and win-lose power struggles with intolerant teachers or inept parents, where the kids almost always lose.

These memories describe an uneven, incoherent set of experiences with Latino and Euro-American mentors. It cannot be assumed that Chicanos will be empathetic or effective mentors, nor that Euro-Americans will be oppressors. What is evident in these quotes is the significance of mentors, particularly Chicano mentors (Romo, 1998), even if they are peers. It is also clear in these memories how I, at various levels of experience, yearned for mentoring, especially when I was the first or second in a particular professional role traditionally held by Euro-Americans.

The interview was a significant event, which helped me to re-invent myself while in relationship to Dr. Marta, a Chicano mentor. I received a different self-image from this elder professional Latino, one that I had not received before. This encounter reflected the power of positive mentoring for me. I looked up to him for his ground breaking form of mentoring. Unfortunately, his direct and confrontational approach about changing the status quo also led to his short term as superintendent. As I reflect on what I have learned from mentors' examples and my ongoing studies (Romo, Bradfield, & Serrano, 2004; Romo & Roseman, 2004), I see activism in three domains: Knowledge, Dispositions (Attitudes, Values, Beliefs) and Skills. These three domains are discussed in the following section.

Knowledge Growth As an Activist: Insights Into Societal Dynamics

Activists appear to embody particular knowledge base, dispositions, and skills related to promoting equity, inclusion and social change

(Romo & Roseman, 2004). The following data represents insights into the theory and practices of racism, classism, and discrimination in general.

For years, I couldn't figure out why some classmates just didn't do as well academically as I did, and I generally thought that it was because I was smarter and that I worked harder than they did. I worked hard to be a perfect student for many years because I held the fantasy that if I were good enough, my dad would stop drinking and our lives would be better. We grew up thinking that we somehow said something or did something that would launch my dad into a rage and drinking spree. Now I know that I wasn't the reason for my dad's outbursts and that it wasn't just my effort that helped me do well in grammar school.

My mother was an avid reader. My father only had a second grade education and often read the newspaper for general information, but my mother read constantly. She never went to college, but she told us that she was an art major in high school, conveying that she had an educational expertise and was proud of what she had done in school and that school was great. From her, my brothers and sisters and I got what lots of middle class kids got, unlike what a lot of poor kids experienced. We had a literature fiend, who used sophisticated vocabulary and developed her social and academic capital farther than her financial capital would ever grow to pass onto her kids. We got her middle class English skills and the benefits of having her at school helping in the office or on field trips. Teachers liked her and us and made us feel valuable and welcome. For lots of poor, Latino kids, school was unwelcoming, disconnected from home language and literacy, and a place of culture shock where finding a gang support system brought more support, acceptance, success and identification than any classroom. I was like the Bre'er Rabbit character in the Uncle Remus story, one of the many stories my mom read to me. School was my briar patch, where I could live well even though lots of my neighborhood kids didn't survive there. Not Sergio Padilla, who got mad at somebody for making fun of his English and went home at lunchtime and brought a butter knife to school to scare his taunter. Not Michael Hubbard (the Mexican kid with the Irish name), who got killed in a drive by. Not Frank Ortega, who struggled in all subjects and faded away long before he stopped coming to school. What might have been their fate if someone had seen their potential and had picked them for something special?

The men who wait and whose souls bleed on corners dream of work and a better life, too. They live in fear of being picked up by the INS, so when sheriff cars drive by, the workers flinch with worry. What will the police do to them, the eternal suspects? I have a taste of that wondering when I get followed by police when I drive my new car, and I wonder if I really did something wrong or is it that my brown face is a magnet for their attention? I wonder because I generally have to show my identification with my local checks, even in local stores I've given patronage to for years—unless I happen to be chatting with a White friend, who the clerk knows. Then, my friend's White face must override my brown face, which somehow makes my check unsafe.

I used to wonder if I was making up this pervasive context of White privilege and hostility towards brown faces. I used to believe those self-proclaimed liberals who said that I was taking things too personally, and that I just needed to lighten up. I now know and my research and extensive conversations with scholars and critical educators from across the nation tell me that the context of White privilege and hostility towards brown faces is pervasive. I see the semi-masked hostility towards brown people beyond the southern California, laid back culture of nice that is distinctive because of our regional economic ties with Mexico. I see that U.S. residents need and hate migrant workers. The need and hate showed itself in the attack in Rancho Penasquitos in the summer of 2000. Several high school White males from a wealthy, 'good' neighborhood hunted and beat elderly brown workers, asleep in their camp in the hills, dreaming of work and a better life. Latino superintendents in my dissertation expressed this conflicted disdain clearly, "'Cause there's people in this community, there's people here at this office who want me to fail. And I know that. I mean, you know that going in: that people want you to fail. Just a matter of life. I mean, they may say to your face, 'Hey, you're doing a great job.' But it makes them ill when they see a Latino running the show." "And I don't care what people tell you, you have some segments of the county here that may talk a good game about minorities, and what they do for 'children of color' but deep in their heart, they're hoping that they'll go away."

In the past, I'd feel like a migrant worker when I stepped out of my set role as a teacher who worked primarily with brown and Asian kids. I once heard the second hand comment, after I had interviewed for an administrative position, that I looked good on paper. That was a code that meant my resume read White, status quo: Stanford B.A., UCLA masters, enrolled at USD in a doctoral program. But my face and soul read migrant.

I knew that coded rejection and it ate at my self-confidence, at my psyche. To protect myself going into interviews, I'd read up on educational research, review interview questions, and listen to spiritual, inspirational tapes. The talks seemed to soothe my ego in advance for the inevitable time that I'd get overly friendly smiles and then hear that someone else with more experience had gotten the job. I was a good candidate; it's just that someone else had more experience. And how the hell was I supposed to get more experience without the job?

For many years, being a migrant professional worker meant going from district to district (I wasn't an insider in my own district). It felt like begging, "Can I work here? Can I do anything here? Can I break my back for you for a day's wage?" I hated that feeling of always looking for a place to call home, a place where I was an insider. Now, I understand the paradox— traveling to find a place as an insider. After five years as a K-12 administrator, I was tired of not seeing my family, of small town educational politics, and of not finishing my doctorate. In my fatigue, I let go of my tentative insider position and I grabbed at the first university job I was offered, thankful to break my back for a day's wage, grateful for a place to work again.

Literacy is an example of the invisible cultural capital that helps students to be successful in school. Without examining how socio-economic status, cultural congruity with schools, social positioning, and other invisible factors that help students feel unskilled or unwanted, meritocracy argues that people are unsuccessful in schools primarily because they don't work hard enough. On the other hand, Freire's (1985) critical pedagogy emphasizes dialogue, praxis (action informed by social justice values), naming the world (e.g., oppression), and a connection with participants' lived experiences. He argued that few human encounters are exempt from oppression because, by virtue of race, class, gender, and ethnicity, people tend to be victims and/or perpetrators of oppression. Freire promoted "problem posing," which integrated theory and practice as a means to clarify the causes and consequences of human suffering. He also advocated this method as a means of developing an ethical and utopian pedagogy for social change.

Critical pedagogy begins with an understanding that knowledge is political and not neutral, and therefore is contextual. Likewise, privilege and authority are political and not neutral. It took years for me to understand that besides my hard work, my mother interjected middle class skills into our home, which gave me access to mainstream curriculum and teaching practices. By understanding white privilege, I can recognize and address its implementation in professional arenas without only taking the experiences as personal insults or attacks. Because I understand identity development processes, I can be more

instructive and effective in mentoring others in their own professional
and personal development processes.

Disposition Growth As an Activist: Victim to Survivor

Educational activists struggle in the everyday to advocate for ALL
students in their ongoing efforts to provide more equitable access to
meaningful challenging educational opportunities. In doing so, they
become aware of their own identities, strengths, and biases and spend
a lifetime reconstructing their own framework of teaching and learning
toward these aims (Romo, Bradfield, & Serrano, 2004). The following
quotes illustrate how discriminatory experiences, once understood in
a societal context, can lead to changes in attitudes, values and beliefs
that support proactive, resilient, and effective advocacy for others.

By that time, I began to see myself as a professional and as others
saw me as less-than professional, I began to speak up. I saw the
dynamic of being seen as 'other' happen in many ways, and once in
a blue moon as an act of kindness. When I was an assistant principal
in another district, I bought and lost a book of stamps at my local post
office. As I retraced my steps a couple of times, searching the premises,
a post office patron met me at the door, pointed to the lettering above
the doorway and loudly enunciated, "POST OFFICE." I actually
laughed and thanked him, instead of challenging him or leaving in a
fury. I knew that this was probably a more polite, albeit patronizing,
version of the old barrio question, "Where are you from?" That simple
misunderstanding articulated a White privilege corollary, toxic
politeness, at work: "You're not from here. You poor thing. You must
be a migrant worker who doesn't understand where you are."

But I guess that it's better to be seen as less than and offered help
than to be seen as a worker instead of a customer at gas stations,
grocery stores or open markets, regardless of what I wear or how I'm
interacting with others. "Could you go in the back and get some more
milk?" I've been asked when I shopped with my daughter, who sat in
the shopping cart. "Could you get the gas?" I've been ordered when
I was wearing my dress slacks, shirt, shoes and tie and pumping my
own gas. "How much are these flowers?" or "Oh, your English is very
good" have come from customers as I stop with my children in front
of a flower stand at our local farmers' market. After a while, I grew
some roots, support and voice. I grew some integrity that told me that
I didn't need others from a district office or committee to validate my
skills or potential to contribute to an organization. When I discovered

that I knew what I knew and that it was valuable and special, I began to speak up and speak out. I began to write books when I began to figure out my life and when I began to read the world itself. It was then that being a migrant professional took on a different life or meaning. I began to go beyond my traditional instinct to wait respectfully and humbly for those in authority to tap me for work or to honor my skills and potential. I had lived in mainstream U.S.A. and had been socialized in educational settings for thirty years, so I believed that hard work and talent alone brought recognition, promotion, and success. Even when I tired of waiting for recognition, it was a major, conscious, counter-intuitive step to go against my cultural trust in humildad or self-deprecation, and to promote myself as a diversity expert, a teacher of teachers and an educational trainer of trainers.

Even though lots of White people positioned me as less-than on a daily basis, I committed to my educational preparation. My master's and doctoral degrees were rites of passage for me. My love of learning brought me back to being a student, but my understanding of where I have come from helped me endure the schedule of teaching or working as an administrator full-time and taking classes at night. I studied for Sergio Padilla, Michael Hubbard and Frank Ortega, for my neighborhood, and for brown kids who didn't survive the educational briar patch. I became driven to change the educational system and society through teacher education. My journey has led me to teach teachers at the university level and at professional conferences.

But now I go against my cultural programming to the police and other groups saying, "I want to work here. I bring valuable expertise that you need to survive in your career. I'm not going away, so let's work together." I put myself in lots of settings knowing that I'll feel the need-hate tension, as an educated, credentialed migrant worker.

Now, I know that if I get followed or stopped [by police], I am not the problem. When I am the usual suspect, an error lies in those who don't even know that they misread me. On the other hand, when I don't get information I need to function smoothly in a new organization, the mistake reflects the problems others have accepting or treating someone they're afraid of with respect. These cultural clashes affect me, but they represent how lots of people don't want to see a brown face take his or her place at the table of legitimacy, decency or authority, as if it would somehow take those privileges away from themselves.

My identity as a migrant worker is redeemed. And my identity, regardless of the setting, is wrapped up in the identities of dark people, especially those who have been used, hurt, marginalized, and minimized. Paulo Freire spoke to my soul when I read that the voices of the marginalized are essential to truly understand and live democracy.

These examples illustrate some of the dispositions (belief in self, valuing self worth) that lead to constructive action. These dispositions grew through risk-taking, doubting, and questioning, and they created and facilitated the conditions for me to find my own voice and participate in transforming my world.

Skill Growth As an Activist: Social Justice/Advocacy Action

Effective activists understand that knowledge itself is political and not neutral, and that schools are a central arena of struggle, resistance, and transformation for both the teacher and the students. They express an appreciation of the forms of tension that open new possibilities of interaction between human beings, and a spirit of challenging the social forces that perpetuate the status quo (Romo, Bradfield, & Serrano, 2004).

When I speak in schools, it's not because I think it's cute or that I think that volunteering is a generally nice idea. It's not even because I know research that highlights the benefits of volunteers, especially those that have expertise that teachers may not have, and shows how volunteers bring role models to students and open up curriculum, etc. I go because now I'm a doctor, an education doctor. I don't wait for the educational disease to grow and manifest itself in later stages; I already see the crisis. We're in an educational emergency and the current practice of letting students go through schools on their own and hopefully end up successful is an abysmal failure.

I go to schools and prescribe developing the strength and forgiveness, not amnesia, to work with those who continue to treat Latinos or others with a need-hate disdain. I also go out to vaccinate: to help people have a sense of warning, a sense of how schools systems in passive and unconscious ways can hurt people, can maim people's identities, can inflict a kind of disease, in a way that the blankets given to Native Americans carried diseases, that then decimate those recipients. This is partly why I teach teachers and why I'm involved with schools. Another reason is that when I look at those at-risk kids, I see myself. I know that through my work, I am redeeming more than schools in general. I am redeeming my own soul. When I see kids who "don't get a second chance . . . who will grab the hand of anybody kind enough to offer it," I see myself. In those moments, I'm the student tadpole keeper, keeper of dreams, keeper of memories of shame and desperate hope in a future mediated by spelling, peeing paradoxes, keeper of a vision of what these student tadpoles can be.

This narrative operationalizes the various themes that the data has identified: addressing cultural capital inequities in schools, mentoring for students of color, presenting positive examples of Chicano leadership to promote a healthy racial identity development, and promoting the positive nature of schools for poor children. I have endeavored to weave accounts of where I have stood as an explanation of where I currently stand as a Chicano activist.[2] My personal and professional growth has not been bounded and stable, but rather bounded by ideals and experiences that surround a dynamic learning process.

Conclusion

This study set out to provide insights into the questions: What factors influence the development of Chicano educational activists? How does Chicano activism in higher education relate to K-12 educational practices for all students? The data suggests that K-12 and university educators should understand themselves and their own identities as members of a team or learning community, as well as the dynamics of isms. They should understand the bittersweet complexities that frame the overall experiences of Chicanos and other students of color in schools. Educators should comprehend the impact of the assimilationist contexts that people of color often experience in schools and in society. To be effective mentors, educators must take into account the discomfort so many Latinos feel about being ethnic in a society that despises Latinos, as well as the desire and fantasy that so many carry to be mainstream. In short, educators must understand the roles they play in many Chicanos' ambivalence about school and authority figures.

It cannot be assumed that Chicanos will be empathetic or effective mentors, nor that Euro-Americans will be oppressors. Advocates for inclusion and equity must examine their own attitudes, values, and beliefs as they relate to helping students develop belief in and valuing of self that lead to constructive action. Activist educators must develop the dispositions that promote student risk-taking, questioning, finding their own voices, and participating in transforming their world. Undergirding educator dispositions is the commitment to all students having a place at the table of academic success.

Educators, therefore, should be able to use an understanding of individual and group motivations and behaviors to create a learning environment that encourages positive social interaction, active engagement in learning, and self-motivation. Educators should be able to bridge the cultural capital expected in mainstream institutions and the experiences of being under-prepared for social or academic rites of passage that many students bring. Educators should be able to facilitate students' negotiating the knowledge, dispositions, and skills from both mainstream and home cultures.

Furthermore, this study suggests that teacher educators and K-12 teachers have many opportunities to promote the inclusion and success of Chicano and other underrepresented students. One immediate systemic reform strategy that emerges from this study is K-12 teachers and teacher educators hear from those who are oppressed by educational systems and advocate for them. Finally, school leaders must act directly to recruit, retain, and mentor Latino and other 'minority' leaders (or those dominant culture members who are biculturally competent) to change educational settings towards equity, inclusion, and respect.

Notes

1. Names in this article have been changed, except for my own.
2. One way that I manifest activism in higher education has been through establishing formal mentor networks. My effort to create the Chicano/Latino Faculty Staff Association in my university (http://www.sandiego.edu/clfsa) and being a spokesperson for the San Diego S.N.A.P. (http://www.snapnetwork.org/) are examples of this activism.

References

Anyon, J. (1980a). Elementary Schooling and the Distinctions of Social Class. *Interchange, 12:* 118–32.

Anyon, J. (1980b). Social Class and the Hidden Curriculum of Work. *Journal of Social Education 16*(2): 1.

Anyon, J. and W. J. Wilson (1997) *Ghetto Schooling: A Political Economy of Urban Educational Reform.* NY, Teachers College Press.

Atkinson, D. R., Morten, G., & Sue, D.W. (Eds.) (1989). *Counseling American minorities: A cross-cultural perspective* (3rd ed.). Dubuque, Iowa: William C. Brown.

Bochner, A. P. (1997). It's about time: Narrative and the divided self. *Qualitative Inquiry, 3*(4): 418–438.

Books, S. (1994). Blaming Villains: Stories of Displacement and Disengagement. *Educational Foundations 8*(3): 5–16.

Bourdieu, P. (1977). Cultural reproduction and social reproduction. In J. Karabel & A. H. Halsey (Eds.), *Power and ideology in education* (pp. 487–511). New York: Oxford University Press.

Charmaz, K., & Mitchell, R. (1997). The myth of silent authorship: Self, substance, and style in ethnographic writing. In R. Hertz, (Ed.), *Reflexivity and voice* (pp. 193–215). London: Sage.

Chávez Chávez, R. (1995). *Multicultural Education for the everyday: A renaissance for the recommitted.* Washington, DC: American Association for Colleges of Teacher Education.

Chávez Chávez, R. (1997). A curriculum discourse for achieving equity: Implications for teachers when engaged with Latina and Latino students. Las Cruces, NM, Unpublished manuscript, New Mexico State University.

Cross, W. E. (1991). *Shades of black: Diversity in African-American identity.* Philadelphia: Temple University Press.

Darder, A., Torres, R. & Gutierrez, H. (Eds.) (1997). *Latinos and education: a critical reader.* New York: Routledge.

Darling-Hammond, L. (1998). Teachers and Teaching: Testing Policy Hypotheses From a National Commission Report. *Educational Researcher 27* (1): 5–15.

Delpit, L. (1995). *Other people's children: Cultural Conflict in the classroom.* NY: New Press.

Edelman, M.W. (1992). *The Measure of Our Success: A Letter to My Children and Yours.* Boston: Beacon Press.

The Education Trust (1998). Thinking K-16. Summer, 3(2): 6.

Ellis, C. & Bochner, A. P. (2000). Autoethnography, personal narrative, reflexivity: Researcher as subject. In N.K. Denzin & Y.S. Lincoln (Eds.) *Handbook of qualitative research* (pp. 733–768). Thousand Oaks, CA: Sage.

Elmore, R.E., & Burney, D. (1997). Investing in teacher learning: Staff development and instructional improvement in Community School District #2, New York City. National Commission on Teaching and America's Future and the Consortium for Policy Research in Education.

Fredrickson, J. (Ed.), (1995). *Reclaiming our voices: Bilingual education, critical pedagogy and praxis.* Ontario: California Association for Bilingual Education.

Freire, P. (1985). *A Pedagogy of the Oppressed.* New York: Continuum Press.

Gonzalez, K, Figueroa, M., Matin, P., Moreno, J., Perez, L. & Navia, C. (1998). Understanding the Nature and Context of Latina/o Doctoral Student Experiences. *Journal of College Student Development, 42*(6): 563–579.

Gonzalez, K., Stone, C., & Jovel, J. (2003) Examining the Role of Social Capital in Access to College for Latinas: Toward a College Opportunity Framework. *Journal of Hispanic Higher Education,* Vol. 2, No. 1, January, pp. 146–170.

Hardiman, R. (1982). White identity development: A process oriented model for describing the racial consciousness of white Americans. Unpublished doctoral dissertation, University of Massachusetts, Amherst.

Haro, R. (1995). Held to a Higher Standard: Latino Executive Selection in Higher Education. In *The leaning ivory tower: Latino professors in American Universities* (Padilla, R. and Chávez Chávez, R., Eds.). New York: State University of New York Press, pp. 189–207.

Helms, J. E. (1990). *Black and White racial identity: Theory, research and practice.* Westport, CT, Greenwood.

Haycock, K. (1997). *Achievement in America.* Washington D.C.: The Education Trust.

Holt, N. (2003). Representation, legitimation, and autoethnography: An autoethnographic writing story. *International Journal of Qualitative Methods,* 2(1). Article 2. Retrieved January 11, 2004 from http://www.ualberta.ca/& sim;iiqm/backissues/2_1/htmt/holt.html

Howard, G. R. (1999). *We Can't Teach What We Don't Know.* New York, Teachers College Press.

Kim, J. (1981). *Process of Asian-American identity development: A study of Japanese American women's perceptions of their struggle to achieve positive identities.* Amherst, MA, University of Massachusetts.

Kitchen, R. S., Velasquez, D.T., & Myers, J. (April, 20001). Dropouts in New Mexico: Native American and Hispanic Students Speak Out. Paper presented at the Annual Meeting of the American Educational Research Association, New Orleans, LA.

Kohl, H. (1994). *"I won't learn from you."* NY, New Press.

McIntosh, P. (1989). White Privilege: Unpacking the invisible knapsack. *Peace and Freedom* 49(4): 10–12.

McLaren, P. (1994). *Life in Schools: An Introduction to Critical Pedagogy in the Foundations of Education.* New York: Longman.

McDermott, P. C. & J. J. Rothenberg (1999). Teaching in High Poverty, Urban Schools—Learning from Practitioners and Students. Annual Meeting of the American Educational Research Association, Montreal, Quebec, Canada.

McDermott, P. & J. Rothenberg (2000). The Characteristics of Effective Teachers in High Poverty Schools—Triangulating Our Data. New Orleans, LA, EDRS.

Moll, L., Gonzales, N., Floyd-Tenery, M., Rivera, A., Rendon, P., Gonzalez, R., & Amanti, C. (1993). Teacher research on funds of knowledge: Learning from households. No. 6. National Center for Research on Cultural Diversity and Second Language Learning.

Moses, R. (2001). *Radical equations: math literacy and civil rights.* Boston: Beacon Press.

Nieto, S. 2000. *Affirming Diversity: The Sociopolitical Context of Multicultural Education.* 3rd ed. Norwell, Mass.: Longman: Addison & Wesley.

Payne, R. K. (1998). A Framework for Understanding Poverty, RFT Publishing Co. Small Schools Workshop, (2001). http://www.smallschools.com/index.html.

Poston, W.S.C. (1990). The biracial identity development model: A needed addition. *Journal of Counseling and Development, 69*: 152–155.

Reed-Danahay, D. (1997). *Auto/Ethnography.* New York: Berg.

Romo, J. (1998). Voices Against Discrimination and Exclusion: Latino School Leaders' Narratives for Change. Unpublished dissertation. University of San Diego.

Romo, J. Bradfield, P. & Serrano, R. (2004). *Reclaiming Democracy: Multicultural Educators' Journeys toward Transformative Teaching*. Cincinnati: Prentice Hall.

Romo, J. & Roseman, M. (2004). In Hughes, L. (Ed.) *Current Issues in Education*. Boston: Lawrence Erlbaum, Inc.

Scheurich, J. J. 1993. Toward a White Discourse on White Racism. *Educational Researcher*. November: 5–10.

Scheurich, J. J. & Young, M. D. (1997). Coloring Epistemologies in Educational Research. *Educational Researcher, 26*(4): 4–16.

Sleeter, C. E., & McLaren, P. L. (Eds.).(1995). *Multicultural education, critical pedagogy, and the politics of difference*. Albany, NY: SUNY Press.

Solis, A. (1981). Theory of biculturality. *Calmecac de Aztlan en Los, 2*: 36–41.

Stanton-Salazar, R.D. (1997). A Social Capital Framework for Understanding the Socialization of Racial Minority Children and Youths. *Harvard Educational Review, 67*(1): 1–41.

Stanton-Salazar, R. D. (2001) *Manufacturing hope and despair: The school and kin support networks of U.S. Mexican youth*. New York: Teachers College Press.

Stonequist, E.V. (1961). *The marginal man: A study in personality and culture conflict*. New York: Russell & Russell, Inc. (Original work published 1937).

Tatum, B. (1998). *Why are all the black kids sitting in the cafeteria?* NY, Perseus Book Company.

Tierney, W. G. (1998). Life history's history: Subjects foretold. *Qualitative Inquiry, 4*, 49–70.

Valenzuela, A. (1999). *Subtractive schooling: U.S.-Mexican youth and the politics of caring*. New York: State University of New York Press.

(Note: Typos from the original print are corrected for this publication.)

NOTES

Chapter 1

1. Triandis (1995) defined collectivism as "a social pattern consisting of closely linked individuals who see themselves as parts of one or more collectives (family, co-workers, tribe, nation); are primarily motivated by the norms of, and duties imposed by, those collectives; are willing to give priority to the goals of these collectives over their own personal goals; and emphasize their connectedness to members of these collectives" (p. 2). Collectivism is contrasted with individualism, defined as "a social pattern that consists of loosely linked individuals who view themselves as independent of collectives; are primarily motivated by their own preferences, needs, rights, and the contracts they have established with others; give priority to their personal goals over the goals of others; and emphasize rational analyses of the advantages and disadvantages to associating with others" (p. 2).
2. Both terms—socialization and enculturation—have been used interchangeably by sociologists and anthropologists. The former term, preferred by sociologists, focuses more on social aspects of becoming a conforming member of a society whereas the latter, preferred by anthropologists, emphasizes learning cultural elements in becoming part of a cultural community.
3. Cultural incongruity, discontinuity, and inconsistency have been written on extensively to describe the cultural differences between minority students' home culture and school culture (Au & Jordan, 1981; Delgado-Gaitan, 1987; Irvine & Armento, 2001; Ladson-Billings, 1994; Mehan, 1987;

Philips, 1983). These concepts are useful in describing the cultural similarities and differences between self and others.

Chapter 3

1. Ellis and Bochner (2000) provide source information for each label.
2. Earlier versions of this section and the next, "Benefits of Autoethnography," and "Pitfalls to Avoid in Doing Autoethnography," were published as part of a chapter, "Autoethnography: Raising Cultural Consciousness of Self and Others," in an edited book by Geoffrey Walford (Chang, 2007).

Chapter 4

1. Although not claimed as an autoethnography, Mead's (1972) autobiography reflects her anthropological insight. The thick description and cultural analysis of her life events add an autoethnographic quality to her life story.

Chapter 8

1. Many commercially developed computer software programs, such as Ethnograph™ or NUD*IST™, are readily available to assist qualitative and ethnographic data analysis.

Chapter 9

1. Wolcott (1994) provided a list of useful data analysis and interpretation strategies for qualitative research. I am borrowing his format here.
2. Microculture, synonymous with subculture, is defined as "a whole way of life culture found within a larger, often complex, society" according to McCurdy, Spradley, and Shandy (2005, p. 14).

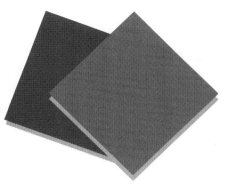

REFERENCES

Achebe, C. (1994). *Things fall apart*. New York: Anchor Books.

Ackerley, J. R. (1975). *My father and myself*. New York: Harcourt Brace Jovanovich.

Adams, H. (2007). *The education of Henry Adams: A centennial version* (Ed., E. Chalfant & C. E. Wright). Boston: Massachusetts Historical Society. (Original published in 1918)

Agar, M. (2006). Culture: Can you take it anywhere? *International Journal of Qualitative Methods, 5*(2), Article 11. Retrieved April 24, 2007, from http://www.ualberta.ca/~iiqm/backissues/5_2/html/agar.htm

Ahmedi, F., & Ansary, T. (2005). *The story of my life: An Afghan girl on the other side of the sky*. New York: Simon Spotlight Entertainment.

Albright, M. (2003). *Madam secretary: A memoir*. New York: The Easton Press.

Allende, I. (2003). *My invented country: A nostalgic journey through Chile* (M. S. Peden, Trans.). New York: HarperCollins.

Anderson, B. G. (2000). *Around the world in 30 years: Life as a cultural anthropologist*. Prospect Heights, IL: Waveland.

Anderson, L. (2006). Analytic autoethnography. *Journal of Contemporary Ethnography, 35*(4), 373–395.

American Heritage Dictionary of the English language (4th ed.). (2000). Boston: Houghton Mifflin.

Angelou, M. (1969). *I know why the caged bird sings*. New York: Random House.

Angrosino, M. V. (Ed.) (2007). *Doing cultural anthropology* (2nd ed.). Long Grove, IL: Waveland.

Armstrong, K. (2005). *Through the narrow gate: A memoir of spiritual discovery*. New York: St. Martin's Griffin.

Atkinson, P. (2006). Rescuing autoethnography. *Journal of Contemporary Ethnography, 35*(4), 400–404.

Asher, N. (2001). Beyond "cool" and "hip": Engaging the question of research and writing as academic self—woman of color other. *International Journal of Qualitative Studies in Education, 14*(1), 1–12.

Attard, K., & Armour, K. M. (2005). Learning to become a learning professional: Reflections on one year of teaching. *European Journal of Teacher Education, 28*(2), 195–207.

Au, K. H., & Jordan, C. (1981). Teaching reading to Hawaiian children: Finding a culturally appropriate solution. In E. T. Trueba, G. P. Guthrie, & K. H. Au (Eds.), *Culture and the bilingual classroom: Studies in classroom ethnography* (pp. 139–152). Rowley, MA: Newbury House Publishers.

Austin, D. A. (1996). Kaleidoscope. In C. Ellis & A. P. Bochner (Eds.), *Composing ethnography: Alternative forms of qualitative writing* (pp. 206–230). Walnut Creek, CA: AltaMira Press.

Azoulay, K. G. (1997). *Black, Jewish, and interracial: It's not the color of your skin, but the race of your kin, and other myths of identity.* Durham, NC: Duke University.

Baker, D. G. (2001). Future homemakers and feminist awakenings: Auto-ethnography as a method in theological education and research. *Religious Education, 96*(3), 395–407.

Baker, R. (1982). *Growing up.* New York: Congdon & Weed.

Baldwin, J. (1963). *Notes of a native son.* New York: Dial Press.

Bates, D. G., & Fratkin, E. M. (2003). *Cultural anthropology* (3rd ed.). Boston: Pearson.

Bateson, M. C. (1994). *With a daughter's eye: A memoir of Margaret Mead and Gregory Bateson.* New York: HarperPerennial.

———— (1995). *Peripheral visions: Learning along the way.* New York: HarperCollins.

Benedict, R. (1934). *Patterns of culture.* New York: Houghton Mifflin.

———— (1946). *The chrysanthemum and the sword.* Cleveland, OH: Meridian Books.

Bepko, C. (1997). *The heart's progress: A memoir.* New York: Penguin Books.

Berger, L. (2007). Messianic Judaism: Searching the spirit. In M. V. Angrosino (Ed.), *Doing cultural anthropology* (pp. 172–174). Long Grove, IL: Waveland.

Berger, L., & Ellis, C. (2007). Composing ethnographic stories. In M. V. Angrosino (Ed.), *Doing cultural anthropology* (2nd ed.) (pp. 161–176). Long Grove, IL: Waveland.

Berry, K. (2006). Implicated audience member seeks understanding: Reexamining the "gift" of autoethnography. *International Journal of Qualitative Methods, 5*(3), Article 7. Retrieved January 26, 2007 from http://www.ualberta.ca/~iiqm/backissues/5_3/pdf/berry.pdf

Best, J. (2006). What, we worry?: The pleasures and costs of defective memory for qualitative sociologists. *Journal of Contemporary Ethnography, 35*(4), 466–478.

Best, J. W., & Kahn, J. V. (2003). *Research in education* (9th ed.). Boston: Pearson Education.

Bochner, A. P., & Ellis, C. (1996). Introduction: Talking over ethnography. In C. Ellis, & A. P. Bochner (Eds.), *Composing ethnography: Alternative forms of qualitative writing* (pp. 13–48). Walnut Creek, CA: AltaMira Press.

Bochner, A. P., & Ellis, C. (Eds.). (2002). *Ethnographically speaking: Auto-ethnography, literature, and aesthetics.* Walnut Creek, CA: AltaMira Press.

Bogdan, R. C., & Biklen, S. K. (2003). *Qualitative research for education: An introduction to theories and methods* (4th ed.). Boston: Allyn and Bacon.

Brayboy, B. M. J. (2005). Transformational resistance and social justice: American Indians in Ivy League universities. *Anthropology and Education Quarterly, 36*(3), 193–211.

Brettell, C. (1997). Blurred genres and blended voices: Life history, biography, autobiography, and the auto/ethnography of women's lives. In D. E. Reed-Danahay (Ed.), *Auto/ethnography: Rewriting the self and the social* (pp. 223–246). New York: Berg.

Breyer, C. (2000). *The close: A young woman's first year at seminary.* New York: Basic Books.

Brookfield, S. D. (1995). *Becoming a critically reflective teacher.* San Francisco: Jossey-Bass.

Brooks, R. (2000). *Blowing Zen: Finding an authentic life.* Tiburon, CA: HJ Kramer.

Brunner, D. D. (1994). *Inquiry and reflection: Framing narrative practice in education.* Albany, NY: SUNY.

Bryant, C. (2007). Planning and moderating focus group research. In M. V. Angrosino (Ed.), *Doing cultural anthropology* (pp. 115–128). Long Grove, IL: Waveland.

Burnier, D. (2006). Encounters with the self in social science research. *Journal of Contemporary Ethnography, 35*(4), 410–418.

Canales, M. K. (2000). Othering: Toward an understanding of difference. *Advances in Nursing Science, 22*(4), 16–31.

Carter, J. (1996). *Living faith.* New York: Times Books.

Cotanda, D. (2006). Voices at mother's kitchen: An autoethnographic account of exile. *Qualitative Inquiry, 12*(3), 562–588.

Chang, H. (1992a). *Adolescent life and ethos: An ethnography of a US high school.* London: Falmer.

——— (1992b). Persist or perish in the qualitative studies of adolescents: Strategies to win a silent negotiation. *1992 QUIG Conference Proceedings.* Athens: University of Georgia.

——— (1999). Cultural autobiography: A tool to multicultural discovery of self. *Electronic Magazine of Multicultural Education, 1*(1). Retrieved December 8, 2005, from http://www.eastern.edu/publications/emme/1999spring/chang.html

——— (2005). Cultural autobiography for Christian multicultural educators: A way of understanding self and others. *A Journal of the International Community of Christians in Teacher Education, 1*(1). Retrieved December 8,

2005, from http://www.icctejournal.org/ICCTEJournal/past_issues/vol1issue1/v1i1chang

Chang, H. (2007). Autoethnography: Raising cultural awareness of self and others. In G. Walford (Ed.). *Studies in educational ethnography Volume 12: Methodological developments in ethnography* (pp. 201–221). Boston: Elsevier.

Chagnon, N. A. (1968). *Yanomamö: The fierce people.* New York: Holt, Rinehart, and Winston.

Chin, E. (2006). Confessions of a negrophile. *Transforming Anthropology, 14*(1), 44–52.

Clandinin, D. J., & Connelly, F. M. (2000). *Narrative inquiry: Experience and story in qualitative research.* San Francisco: Jossey-Bass.

Clausen, C., & Cruickshank, D. R. (1991). *Reflective teaching.* Columbus: Ohio State University.

Clifford, J., & Marcus, G. (Eds.). (1986). *Writing culture: The poetics and politics of ethnography.* Berkeley: University of California.

Clinton, B. (2004). *My life.* New York: Knopf.

Clinton, H. R. (2004). *Living history.* New York: Scribner.

Coia, L., & Taylor, M. (2006). From the inside out and the outside in: Co/autoethnography as a means of professional renewal. In C. Kosnik *et al.* (Eds.), *Making a difference in teacher education through self-study* (pp. 19–33). Amsterdam: Springer.

Corse, S. J. (2004). *Cradled all the while: The unexpected gifts of a mother's death.* Minneapolis, MN: Augsburg Books.

Crane, C. (2000). *Divided lives: The untold stories of Jewish-Christian women in Nazi Germany.* New York: Palgrave Macmillan.

Crapanzano, V. (1980). *Tuhami: Portrait of a Moroccan.* Chicago: University of Chicago.

Creswell, J. W. (1998). *Qualitative inquiry and research design: Choosing among five traditions.* Thousand Oaks, CA: Sage.

——— (2002). *Research design: Qualitative, quantitative, and mixed methods approaches* (2nd ed.). Thousand Oaks, CA: Sage.

Crossan, J. D. (2000). *A long way from Tipperary.* San Francisco: HarperSan Francisco.

De Beauvoir, S. (2005). *Memoirs of a dutiful daughter.* New York: Harper Perennial.

De Munck, V. (2000). *Culture, self, and meaning.* Prospect Heights, IL: Waveland Press.

Delgado-Gaitan, C. (1987). Traditions and transitions in the learning process of Mexican children: An ethnographic view. In G. D. Spindler & L. Spindler, (Eds.). *Interpretive ethnography of education: At home and abroad* (pp. 333–362). Hillsdale, NJ: L. Erlbaum Associates.

Denzin, N. (1997). *Interpretive ethnography: Ethnographic practices for the 21st century.* Thousand Oaks, CA: Sage.

——— (2003). The call to performance. *Symbolic Interaction, 26*(1), 187–207.

——— (2006). Analytic autoethnography, or déjà vu all over again. *Journal of Contemporary Ethnography, 35*(4), 419–428.

Denzin, N. K., & Lincoln, Y. S., (Eds.). (1994). *Handbook of qualitative research.* Thousands Oaks, CA: Sage.

———— (Eds.). (2000). *Handbook of qualitative research* (2nd ed.). Thousand Oaks, CA: Sage.

deRoche, C. P. (2007). Exploring genealogy. In M. V. Angrosino (Ed.), *Doing cultural anthropology* (pp. 19–32). Long Grove, IL: Waveland.

Dillard, A. (1987). *An American childhood.* New York: Harper & Row.

Donofrio, B. (2000). *Looking for Mary (or, the Blessed Mother and me).* New York: Viking Compass.

Douglass, F. (1995). *Narrative of the life of Frederick Douglass.* New York: Dover Publications.

Dubner, S. J. (1999). *Turbulent souls: A Catholic son's return to his Jewish family.* New York: Avon Books.

Dubus, A. (1998). *Meditations from a movable chair.* New York: Alfred A. Knopf.

Duckart, T. (2005). Autoethnography. Retrieved September 20, 2005, from http://www.humboldt.edu/~tdd2/Autoethnography.htm

Edelman, M. (1996). Devil, not-quite-White, rootless cosmopolitan *Tsuris* in Latin America, the Bronx, and the USSR. In C. Ellis & A. P. Bochner (Eds.), *Composing ethnography: Alternative forms of qualitative writing* (pp. 267–300). Walnut Creek, CA: AltaMira Press.

Edelman, M. W. (1999). *Lanterns: A memoir of mentors.* New York: HarperCollins.

Ellis, C. (1995). *Final negotiations: A story of love, loss, and chronic illness.* Philadelphia: Temple University.

———— (1996). Maternal connections. In C. Ellis & A. P. Bochner (Eds.), *Composing ethnography: Alternative forms of qualitative writing* (pp. 240–243). Walnut Creek, CA: AltaMira Press.

———— (2004). *The ethnographic I: A methodological novel about autoethnography.* Walnut Creek, CA: AltaMira Press.

Ellis, C., & Bochner, A. P. (Eds.) (1996). *Composing ethnography: Alternative forms of qualitative writing.* Walnut Creek, CA: AltaMira Press.

Ellis, C. S., & Bochner, A. P. (2000). Autoethnography, personal narrative, and personal reflexivity. In N. K. Denzin & Y. S. Lincoln (Eds.), *Handbook of qualitative research* (2nd ed.) (pp. 733–768). Thousand Oaks, CA: Sage.

———— (2006). Analyzing analytic autoethnography. *Journal of Contemporary Ethnography, 35*(4), 429–449.

Ellis, C., & Flaherty, M. G. (1992). *Investigating subjectivity: Research on lived experience.* Thousand Oaks, CA: Sage.

Erickson, F. (2004). Culture in society and in educational practices. In J. A. Banks & C. A. M. Banks (Eds.), *Multicultural education: Issues and perspectives* (5th ed.) (pp. 31–60). Hoboken, NJ: John Wiley & Sons.

Ettorre, E. (2005). Gender, older female bodies and autoethnography: Finding my feminist voice by telling my illness story. *Women's Studies International Forum, 28*(6), 535–546.

Florio-Ruane, S. (2001). *Teacher education and the cultural imagination.* Mahwah, NJ: Lawrence Erlbaum.

Foltz, T. G., & Griffin, W. (1996). She changes everything she touches: Ethnographic journeys of self-discovery. In C. Ellis & A. P. Bochner (Eds.), *Composing ethnography: Alternative forms of qualitative writing* (pp. 301–329). Walnut Creek, CA: AltaMira Press.

Fontana, A., & Frey, J. H. (2000). The interview: From structured questions to negotiated text. In N. K. Denzin & Y. S. Lincoln (Eds.), *Handbook of qualitative research* (2nd ed.) (pp. 645–672). Thousand Oaks, CA: Sage.

Foster, K., McAllister, M., & O'Brien, L. (2005). Coming to autoethnography: A mental health nurse's experience. *International Journal of Qualitative Methods, 4*(4), Article 1. Retrieved June 30, 2006, from http://www.ualberta.ca/~iiqm/backissues/4_4/html/foster.htm

Fox, K. V. (1996). Silent voices: A subversive reading of child sexual abuse. In C. Ellis & A. P. Bochner (Eds.), *Composing ethnography: Alternative forms of qualitative writing* (pp. 330–356). Walnut Creek, CA: AltaMira Press.

Frankenberg, R. (1993). *White women, race matters: The social construction of whiteness.* Minneapolis: University of Minnesota.

Freeman, M. (2004). Data are everywhere: Narrative criticism in the literature of experience. In C. Dauite & C. Lightfoot (Eds.), *Narrative analysis: Studying the development of individuals in society* (pp. 63–82). Thousand Oaks, CA: Sage.

Fries, K. (Ed.). (1997). *Staring back: The disability experience from the inside out.* New York: A Plum Book.

Gajjala, R. (2004). *Cyber selves.* Walnut Creek, CA: AltaMira Press.

Gallas, K. (1998). *Sometimes I can be anything: Power, gender, and identity in a primary classroom.* New York: Teachers College.

Gandhi, M. (1957). *Autobiography: The story of my experiments with the truth.* Boston: Beacon.

Gatson, S. N. (2003). On being amorphous: Autoethnography, genealogy, and a multiracial identity. *Qualitative Inquiry, 9*(1), 20–48.

Geertz, C. (1973). *The interpretation of cultures.* New York: Basic Books.

―――― (1984). From the native's point of view: On the nature of anthropological understanding. In R. A. Shweder & R. A. Levine (Eds.), *Culture theory: Essays on mind, self, and emotion* (pp. 123–136). Cambridge, UK: Cambridge University.

―――― (1995). *After the fact: Two centuries, four decades, one anthropologist.* Cambridge, MA: Harvard University.

Gergen, K. J. (1991). *The saturated self: Dilemmas of identity in contemporary life.* New York: Basic Books.

Gergen, M., & Gergen, K. (2002). Ethnographic representation as relationship. In A. Bochner & C. Ellis (Eds.), *Ethnographically speaking: Autoethnography, literature, and aesthetics* (pp. 11–33). Walnut Creek, CA: AltaMira Press.

Gilbert, O., with Sojourner Truth. (1997). *Narrative of Sojourner Truth.* Mineola, NY: Dover.

Goldberg, N. (1993). *Long quiet highway.* New York: Bantam Books.

Goldschmidt, W. (1977). Anthropology and the coming crisis: An autoethnographic appraisal. *American Anthropologist, 79*(2), 293–308.

Goodenough, W. (1976). Multiculturalism as the normal human experience. *Anthropology and Education Quarterly, 7*(4), 4–7.

———— (1981). *Culture, language, and society.* Menlo Park, CA: The Benjamin/ Cummings Publishing Company.

Gornick, V. (2001). *The situation and the story: The art of personal narrative.* New York: Farrar, Straus & Giroux.

Greene, M. (2000). The passions of pluralism: Multiculturalism and the expanding community. In J. Noel (Ed.), *Sources: Notable selection in multicultural education* (pp. 38–46). Guilford, CT: Dushkin/McGraw-Hill.

Grenz, S. J. (1996). *A primer on postmodernism.* Grand Rapids, MI: William B. Eerdmans Publishing Company.

Haley, A., & Malcolm X. (1996). *The autobiography of Malcolm X.* New York: Chelsea House Publishers.

Hall, E. T. (1973). *The silent language: An anthropologist reveals how we communicate by our manners and behavior.* Garden City, NY: Anchor Books.

Halverson, C. (2004). *Maverick autobiographies: Women writers and the American West 1900–1936.* Madison: University of Wisconsin.

Harper, D. (2000). Reimagining visual methods: Galileo to *Neuromancer.* In N. K. Denzin & Y. S. Lincoln (Eds.), *Handbook of qualitative research* (2nd ed.) (pp. 717–732). Thousand Oaks, CA: Sage.

Harris, M. (1975). *Culture, people, and nature: An introduction to general anthropology* (2nd ed.). New York: Harper International.

Hathaway, J. (1992). *Motherhouse.* New York: Hyperion.

Hayano, D. M. (1979). Auto-Ethnography: Paradigms, problems, and prospects. *Human Organization, 38*(1), 99–104.

———— (1982). *Poker faces: The life and work of professional card players.* Berkeley: University of California.

Heider, K. G. (1975). What do people do? Dani auto-ethnography. *Journal of Anthropological Research, 31,* 3–17.

Herrmann, A. F. (2005). My father's ghost: Interrogating family photos. *Journal of Loss & Trauma, 10*(4), 337–346.

Hodder, I. (2003). The interpretation of documents and material culture. In N. K. Denzin and Y. S. Lincoln (Eds.), *Collecting and interpreting qualitative materials* (2nd ed.), (pp. 155–175). Thousand Oaks, CA: Sage.

Hoffman, D. M. (1996). Culture and self in multicultural education: Reflections on discourse, text, and practice. *American Educational Research Journal, 33*(3), 545–569.

Holt, N. L. (2003). Representation, legitimation, and autoethnography: An autoethnographic writing story. *International Journal of Qualitative Methods, 2*(1). Retrieved March 13, 2006, from http://www.ualberta.ca/~iiqm/ backissues/2_1final/html/holt.html

Humphreys, M. (2005). Getting personal: Reflexivity and autoethnographic vignettes. *Qualitative Inquiry, 11*(6), 840–860.

Hurston, Z. N. (1984). *Dust tracks on a road.* Urbana: University of Illinois.

Ikeda, K. (1998). *A room full of mirrors: High school reunions in middle America.* Stanford, CA: Stanford University.

Irvine, J. J., & Armento, B. J. (2001). *Culturally responsive teaching: Lesson planning for elementary and middle grades.* New York: McGraw Hill.

Jamison, K. R. (1996). *An unquiet mind.* New York: Vintage Books.

Kaplan, D., & Manners, R. A. (1972). *Culture theory.* Prospect Heights, IL: Waveland.

Keesing, R. (1976). *Cultural anthropology: A contemporary perspective.* New York: Holt, Rinehart and Winston.

Kelley, H., & Betsalel, K. (2004). Mind's fire: Language, power, and representations of stroke. *Anthropology and Humanism, 29*(2), 104–116.

Kempe, M. (2000). *Book of Margery Kempe* (B. Windeatt, Trans.). New York: Penguin Classics.

Kennett, C. L. (1999). Saying more than hello: Creating insightful cross-cultural conversations. In D. C. Elliott & S. D. Holtrop (Eds.), *Nurturing and reflective teachers: A Christian approach for the 21st century* (pp. 229–248). Claremont, CA: Learning Light Educational Consulting and Publishing.

Kidd, S. M. (2002). *The dance of the dissident daughter.* San Francisco: HarperCollins.

Kikumura, A. (1981). *Through harsh winters: The life of a Japanese immigrant woman.* Novato, CA: Chandler & Sharp.

Kim, E. (2000). Korean adoptee auto-ethnography: Refashioning self, family, and finding community. *Visual Anthropology Review, 16*(1), 43–70.

Kingston, M. H. (1989). *The woman warrior.* New York: Vintage Books.

Kitzinger, J. (1999). The methodology of focus groups: The importance of interaction between research participants. In A. Bryman & R. G. Burgess (Eds.), *Qualitative research: Volume II* (pp. 138–155). Thousand Oaks, CA: Sage.

Kreb, N. B. (1999). *Edgewalkers: Defusing cultural boundaries on the new global front.* Far Hills, NJ: New Horizon.

Kroeber, A. L., & Kluckhohn, C. (1966). *Culture: A critical review of concepts and definitions.* New York: Random House. (Originally published in 1952).

Kübler-Ross, E., & Gold, T. (1997). *The wheel of life: A memoir of living and dying.* New York: Scribner.

Ladson-Billings, G. (1994). *The dreamkeepers: Successful teachers of African American children.* San Francisco: Jossey-Bass.

Lamott, A. (2000). *Traveling mercies: Some thoughts on faith.* New York: Anchor Books.

———— (2005). *Plan B: Further thoughts on faith.* New York: Riverhead Hardcover.

Lavery, D. (1999). *Autobiographies: A checklist.* Retrieved April 9, 1999, from http://www.mtsu.edu/~dlavery/abchk.htm

Lazarre, J. (1996). *Beyond the whiteness of whiteness: Memoir of a White mother of Black sons.* Durham, NC: Duke University.

Lee, D. (1959). *Freedom and culture.* Upper Saddle River, NJ: Prentice-Hall.

———— (1986). *Valuing the self: What we can learn from other cultures.* Prospect Heights, IL: Waveland.

Lewis, C. S. (1956). *Surprised by joy.* New York: Harcourt Brace.

———— (1978). *The chronicles of Narnia: The lion, the witch, and the wardrobe.* New York: HarperCollins.

Lightfoot, C. (2004). Fantastic self: A study of adolescents' fictional narratives, and aesthetic activity as identity work. In C. Dauite & C. Lightfoot (Eds.), *Narrative analysis: Studying the development of individuals in society* (pp. 21–38). Thousand Oaks, CA: Sage.

Lingenfelder, J. (1996). Training education students for multicultural classrooms. *Christian Scholar's Review, 25*(4), 491–507.

Lott, B. (1997). *Fathers, sons, and brothers.* New York: Harcourt Brace.

Lucal, B. (1999). What it means to be gendered me: Life on the boundaries of a dichotomous gender system. *Gender and Society, 13*(6), 781–797.

Luke, C. (1994). White women in interracial families: Reflections on hybridization, feminine identities, and racialized othering. *Feminist Issues, 14*(2), 49–72.

MacKie, C. P. (1891). *With the admiral of the ocean sea: A narrative of the first voyage to the western world drawn mainly from the diary of Christopher Columbus.* Chicago: A. C. McClurg and Company.

Madriz, E. (2003). Focus groups in feminist research. In N. K. Denzin & Y. S. Lincoln. (pp. 363–388). *Collecting and interpreting qualitative materials* (2nd ed.). Thousand Oaks, CA: Sage.

Magnet, S. (2006). Protesting privilege: An autoethnographic look at whiteness. *Qualitative Inquiry, 12*(4), 736–749.

Malinowski, B. (1967). *A diary in the strict sense of the term* (N. Guterman, Trans.). New York: Harcourt, Brace, & World.

Mandela, N. (1994). *Long walk to freedom: The autobiography of Nelson Mandela.* London: Little, Brown and Company.

Malina, B. J. (1993). *The New Testament world: Insights from cultural anthropology.* Louisville, KY: Westminster/John Knox.

Mason, M. (1992). Dorothy Day and women's spiritual autobiography. In M. Culley (Ed.), *American women's autobiography: Fea(s)ts of memory* (pp. 185–217). Madison: University of Wisconsin.

Maxwell, J. A. (2005). *Qualitative research design: An interactive approach.* Thousand Oaks, CA: Sage.

McBride, J. (1996). *The color of water: A Black man's tribute to his White mother.* New York: Riverhead Books.

McCurdy, D. W., Spradley, J. P., & Shandy, D. J. (2005). *The cultural experience: Ethnography in complex society* (2nd ed.). Long Grove, IL: Waveland Press.

McKay, N. Y. (1998). The narrative self: Race, politics, and culture in Black American women's autobiography. In S. Smith & J. Watson (Eds.), *Women, autobiography, theory* (pp. 96–107). Madison: University of Wisconsin.

Mead, M. (1972). *Blackberry winter: My earlier years.* New York: Morrow.

—— (1978). *Culture and commitment.* Garden City, NY: Anchor Books.

Mehan, H. (1987). Language and schooling. In G. D. Spindler & L. Spindler, (Eds.). *Interpretive ethnography of education: At home and abroad* (pp. 109–136). Hillsdale, NJ: L. Erlbaum Associates.

Meneses, E. H. (2000). No other foundation: Establishing Christian anthropology. *Christian Scholar's Review, 29*(3), 531–549.

Merton, R. K. (1999). The focused interview and focus groups: Continuities and discontinuities. In A. Bryman & R. G. Burgess (Eds.), *Qualitative research: Volume II* (pp. 122–137). Thousand Oaks, CA: Sage.

Momaday, N. S. (1976). *The names: A memoir.* New York: Harper & Row.

Morse, J. M. (1994). Emerging from the data: The cognitive processes of analysis in qualitative inquiry. In J. M. Morse (Ed.), *Critical issues in qualitative research methods* (pp. 23–43). Thousand Oaks, CA: Sage.

—— (2002). Editorial: Writing my own experience. *Qualitative Health Research, 12*(9), 1159–1160.

Motzafi-Haller, P. (1997). Writing birthright: On native anthropologists and the politics of representation. In D. E. Reed-Danahay, (Ed.), *Auto/ethnography: Rewriting the self and the social* (pp. 195–222). Oxford, UK: Berg.

Muncey, T. (2005). Doing autoethnography. *International Journal of Qualitative Methods, 4*(1). Retrieved Februrary 9, 2006, from http://www.ualberta.ca/~iiqm/backissues/4_1/html/muncey.htm

Nash, R. J. (2002). *Spirituality, ethics, religion, and teaching: A professor's journey.* New York: Peter Lang Publishing.

—— (2004). *Liberating scholarly writing: The power of personal narrative.* New York: Teachers College.

Neumann, M. (1992). The trail through experience: Finding self in the recollection of travel. In C. Ellis & M. G. Flaherty (Eds.). *Investigating subjectivity: Research on lived experience* (pp. 176–201). Thousand Oaks, CA: Sage.

Neville-Jan, A. (2003). Encounters in a world of pain: An autoethnography. *American Journal of Occupational Therapy, 57*(1), 88–98.

Nieto, S. (2003). *What keeps teachers going?* New York: Teachers College.

—— (2004). *Affirming diversity: The sociopolitical context of multicultural education* (4th ed.). Boston: Allyn and Bacon.

Noel, J. (Ed.). (2000). *Sources: Notable selection in multicultural education.* Guilford, CT: Dushkin/McGraw-Hill.

Norris, K. (1996). *Cloister walk.* New York: Riverhead Books.

—— (2001). *Dakota: A spiritual geography.* Boston: Houghton Mifflin.

Obidah, J. E., & Teel, K. M. (2001). *Because of the kids: Facing racial and cultural differences in schools.* New York: Teachers College.

Olson, B. (1993). *Bruchko.* Orlando, FL: Creation House.

Olson, L. N. (2004). The role of voice in the (re)construction of a battered woman's identity: An autoethnography of one woman's experiences of abuse. *Women's Studies in Communication, 27*(1), 1–33.

Ortner, S. B. (2003). *New Jersey dreaming: Capital, culture, and the class of '58.* Durham, NC: Duke University.

Panko, S. M. (1976). *Martin Buber.* Waco, TX: Word Books.

Parks, R. (1992). *Rosa Parks: My story.* New York: Dial Books.

Peterson, M. K. (2003). *Sing me to heaven.* Grand Rapids, MI: Brazos.

Phifer, N. (2002). *Memoirs of the soul.* Cincinnati, OH: Walking Stick Press.

Philips, S. U. (1983). *The invisible culture: Communication in classroom and community on the Warm Springs Indian reservation.* Prospect Heights, IL: Waveland.

Plourde, B. (2005). *Rose of many colors*. Frederick, MD: PublishAmerica.

Pohl, C. D. (1999). *Making room: Recovering hospitality as a Christian tradition*. Grand Rapids, MI: William B. Eerdmans Publishing.

Powell, C., & Persico, J. E. (1995). *My American journey*. New York: Ballantine Books.

Powell, R., Zehm, S., & Garcia, J. (1996). *Field experience: Strategies for exploring diversity in schools*. Upper Saddle River, NJ: Prentice Hall.

Princeton University (2006). Wordnet Search 3.0. Retrieved June 30, 2006, from http://wordnet.princeton.edu/perl/webwn

Peoples, J., & Bailey, G. (2003). *Humanity: An introduction to cultural anthropology*. Belmont, CA: Wadsworth/Thomson.

Quinney, R. (1996). Once my father traveled west to California. In C. Ellis & A. P. Bochner (Eds.). *Composing ethnography: Alternative forms of qualitative writing* (pp. 357–382). Walnut Creek, CA: AltaMira Press.

Radcliffe-Brown, A. R. (1958). *Method in social anthropology: Selected essays*. Chicago: University of Chicago.

Reed-Danahay, D. E. (Ed.). (1997). *Auto/ethnography: Rewriting the self and the social*. Oxford, UK: Berg.

Richardson, L. (1992). The consequences of poetic representation: Writing the other, rewriting the self. In C. Ellis & M. G. Flaherty (Ed.), *Investigating subjectivity: Research on lived experience* (pp. 125–140). Thousands Oaks, CA: Sage.

Rodriguez, N., & Ryave, A. (2002). *Systematic self-observation*. Thousand Oaks, CA: Sage.

Rodriguez, R. (1982). *Hunger of memory: The education of Richard Rodriguez*. New York: Bantam Books.

Romo, J. J. (2004). Experience and context in the making of a Chicano activist. *High School Journal, 87*(4), 95–111.

Ronai, C. R. (1996). My mother is mentally retarded. In C. Ellis & A. P. Bochner (Eds.), *Composing ethnography: Alternative forms of qualitative writing* (pp. 109–131). Walnut Creek, CA: AltaMira Press.

Roosevelt, E. (1984). *The autobiography of Eleanor Roosevelt*. Boston: G.K. Hall.

Rosaldo, M. (1984). Toward an anthropology of self and feeling. In R. A. Shweder & R. A. LeVine (Eds.), *Culture theory: Essays on mind, self, and emotion* (pp. 137–157). Cambridge, UK: Cambridge University.

Rushing, J. H. (2006). *Erotic mentoring: Women's transformations in the university*. Walnut Creek, CA: Left Coast Press.

Sack, R. D. (1997). *Homo geographicus: A framework for action, awareness, and moral concern*. Baltimore, MD: Johns Hopkins University.

Saint Augustine. (1999). *The confessions of St. Augustine*. (E. B. Pusey, Trans.). New York: Barnes and Noble Books.

Salzman, P. C. (2002). On reflexivity. *American Anthropologist, 104*(3), 805–813.

Sands, K. M. (1992). Indian women's personal narrative: Voices past and present. In M. Culley (Ed.), *American women's autobiography* (pp. 268–294). Madison: University of Wisconsin.

Schafer, R. (1992). *Retelling a life: Narrative and dialogue in psychoanalysis*. New York: Basic Books.

Schensul, S. L., Schensul, J. J., & LeCompte, M. D. (1999). *Essential ethnographic methods: Observations, interviews, and questionnaires.* Walnut Creek, CA: AltaMira Press.

Schneider, B. (2005). Mothers talk about their children with schizophrenia: A performance autoethnography. *Journal of Psychiatric & Mental Health Nursing, 12*(3), 333–340.

Schwartz, T. (1978). Where is the culture? Personality as the locus of culture. In G. De Cos (Ed.), *Making of psychological anthropology* (pp. 419–441). Berkeley, CA: University of California.

Shank, G. D. (2002). *Qualitative research: A personal skills approach.* Upper Saddle River, NJ: Merrill Prentice Hall.

Shaw, K. M., Valadez, J. R., & Rhoads, R.A. (Eds.) (1999). *Community colleges as cultural texts: Qualitative explorations of organizational and student culture.* New York: State University of New York.

Silverman, D. (2000). *Doing qualitative research: A practical handbook.* Thousand Oaks, CA: Sage.

Simmons, L. W. (Ed.). (1942). *Sun Chief: An autobiography of a Hopi Indian.* New Haven, CT: Yale University.

Sinopoli, R. C. (Ed.). (1997). *From many, one: Readings in American political and social thoughts.* Washington, DC: Georgetown University.

Smith, C. (2005). Epistemological intimacy: A move to autoethnography. *International Journal of Qualitative Methods, 4*(2), Article 6. Retrieved June 30, 2006, from http://www.ualberta.ca/~iiqm/backissues/4_2/HTML/smith.htm

Sparkes, A. C. (2002). Autoethnography: Self-indulgence or something more? In A. Bochner & C. Ellis (Eds.), *Ethnographically speaking: Autoethnography, literature, and aesthetics* (pp. 209–232). Walnut Creek, CA: AltaMira Press.

Spindler, G. D. (Ed.). (1983). *Being an anthropologist: Fieldwork in eleven cultures.* New York: Irvington Publishers.

Spradley, J. P. (1979). *The ethnographic interview.* New York: Holt, Rinehart and Winston.

Spring, J. (2004). *The intersection of cultures* (3rd ed.). Boston: McGraw Hill.

Stephan, W. G. (1999). *Reducing prejudice and stereotyping in the schools.* New York: Teachers College.

Taber, N. (2005). Learning how to be a woman in the Canadian Forces/unlearning it through feminism: An autoethnography of my learning journey. *Studies in Continuing Education, 27*(3), 289–301.

Taves, A. K. (1992). Self and god in the early published memoirs of New England women. In M. Culley (Ed.), *American women's autobiography: Fea(s)ts of memory* (pp. 57–74). Madison: University of Wisconsin.

Taylor, C. (1989). *Sources of the self: The making of the modern identity.* Cambridge, MA: Harvard University.

Taylor, S. (2005). Identity trouble and opportunity in women's narratives of residence. *Auto/Biography,13,* 249–265.

Taylor, S. J., & Bogdan, R. (1984). *Introduction to qualitative research methods: The search for meanings.* New York: John Wiley & Sons.

Tedlock, B. (2000). Ethnography and ethnographic representation. In N. K. Denzin & Y. S. Lincoln (Eds.), *Handbook of qualitative research* (2nd ed.) (pp. 455–486). Thousand Oaks, CA: Sage.

Thayer-Bacon, B. J., & Bacon, C. S. (1998). *Philosophy applied to education: Nurturing a democratic community in the classroom.* Upper Saddle River, NJ: Merrill.

Thompson, E. P. (1994). *Making history: Writings on history and culture.* New York: W. W. Norton.

Tiedt, P. L., & Tiedt, I. M. (2005). *Multicultural teaching: A handbook of activities, information, and resources* (7th ed.). Boston: Allyn and Bacon.

Tillmann-Healy, L. M. (1996). A secret life in a culture of thinness: Reflections on body, food, and bulimia. In C. Ellis & A. P. Bochner (Eds.), *Composing ethnography: Alternative forms of qualitative writing* (pp. 76–108). Walnut Creek, CA: AltaMira Press.

Tompkins, J. P. (1996). *A life in school: What the teacher learned.* Reading, MA: Perseus Books.

Triandis, H. C. (1995). *Individualism and collectivism.* Boulder, CO: Westview.

Tylor, E. B. (1871). *Primitive culture.* London: J. Murray.

Van Maanen, J. (1988). *Tales of the field: On writing ethnography.* Chicago: University of Chicago.

Vitz, P. C. (1977). *Psychology as religion: The cult of self-worship* (2nd ed.). Grand Rapids, MI: William B. Eerdmans.

Wakefield, D. (1990). *The story of your life: Writing a spiritual autobiography.* Boston: Beacon.

Walker, R. (2001). *Black, White, and Jewish: An autobiography of a shifting self.* New York: Berkley Publishing Group.

Wall, S. (2006). An autoethnography on learning about autoethnography. *International Journal of Qualitative Methods, 5*(2), Article 9. Retrieved January 26, 2007, from http://www.ualberta.ca/~ijqm/backissues/5_2/html/wall.htm

Wolcott, H. F. (1991). Propriospect and the acquisition of culture. *Anthropology and Education Quarterly, 22*(3), 251–273.

——— (1994). *Transforming qualitative data: Description, analysis, and interpretation.* Thousand Oaks, CA: Sage.

——— (2001). *Writing up qualitative research* (2nd ed.). Thousand Oaks, CA: Sage.

——— (2003a). *A Kwakiutl village and school.* Walnut Creek, CA: AltaMira Press.

——— (2003b). *The man in the principal's office.* Walnut Creek, CA: AltaMira Press.

——— (2004). The ethnographic autobiography. *Auto/Biography, 12,* 93–106.

Wyatt, J. (2005). A gentle going? An autoethnographic short story. *Qualitative Inquiry, 11*(5), 724–732.

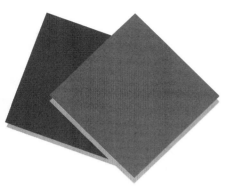

INDEX

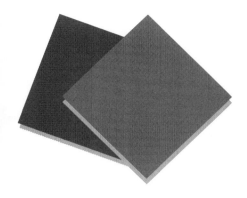

ABOUT THE AUTHOR

Heewon Chang, Ph.D., is Associate Professor of Education at Eastern University in Pennsylvania. Trained as an educational anthropologist, she has conducted ethnographic studies of adolescents in the United States and Korea, one of which was published in *Adolescent Life and Ethos: An Ethnography of a US High School* (1992). While keeping up her interest in the ethnography of adolescents, she has expanded her research focus to autoethnography, multicultural education, cultural identity, and gender issues. She founded two open-access online journals—*Electronic Magazine of Multicultural Education* in 1999 and *International Journal of Multicultural Education* in 2007—and has served on them as Editor-in-Chief. Personally she has embraced Korean, U.S., and German cultures through birth, migration, and marriage. Her multiculturality informs her professional life.